Dear Maria

Lovely meeting a
real-life cheer leader!

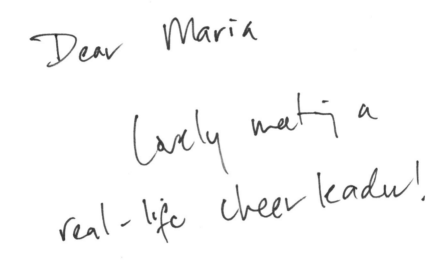

Neuroimaging clearly shows that the female brain has many unique strengths, and in this fascinating book, Tracy Alloway gives women a blueprint to take advantage of that three-pound supercomputer between their ears.

DANIEL G. AMEN, MD, AUTHOR OF *CHANGE YOUR BRAIN, CHANGE YOUR LIFE* AND *YOUR BRAIN IS ALWAYS LISTENING*

Think Like a Girl is a practical and inspiring book, full of groundbreaking insights for women in every field. For readers looking to harness their natural abilities, grow in their confidence, and take leaps forward in their careers or personal lives, this book is an important read!

MARSHALL GOLDSMITH, *NEW YORK TIMES* #1 BESTSELLING AUTHOR OF *TRIGGERS*, *MOJO*, AND *WHAT GOT YOU HERE WON'T GET YOU THERE*

Dr. Alloway's book is not only a call to lean into the very real and beautiful things that make the female brain unique . . . it also lends scientific validity and . . . *permission* to do so, proudly and unabashedly.

KIM CARAMELE, EMMY-WINNING WRITER AND PRODUCER

Dr. Tracy Alloway's new book, *Think Like a Girl*, is a briskly written and engaging account of how women can leverage their unique competencies in ways that promote both personal and professional growth.

ROBERT HOGAN, PHD, PRESIDENT OF HOGAN ASSESSMENTS

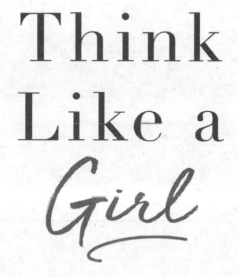

Think
Like a
Girl

Think
Like a
Girl

10 Unique Strengths of a Woman's Brain
and How to Make Them Work for You

Tracy Packiam Alloway, PhD

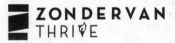

ZONDERVAN
THRIVE

ZONDERVAN THRIVE

Think Like a Girl
Copyright © 2021 by Tracy Alloway

Requests for information should be addressed to:
Zondervan, *3900 Sparks Dr. SE, Grand Rapids, Michigan 49546*

Zondervan titles may be purchased in bulk for educational, business, fundraising, or sales promotional use. For information, please email SpecialMarkets@Zondervan.com.

ISBN 978-0-310-36314-9 (international trade paper edition)
ISBN 978-0-310-36122-0 (audio)

Library of Congress Cataloging-in-Publication Data

Names: Alloway, Tracy Packiam, author.
Title: Think like a girl : 10 unique strengths of a woman's brain and how to make them work for you / Tracy Packiam Alloway.
Description: Grand Rapids : Zondervan, 2021. | Includes bibliographical references. | Summary: "In Think Like a Girl, award-winning psychologist, researcher, and TEDx speaker Dr. Alloway presents powerful myth-busting research about how the female brain is different, why this matters, and ten tactical ways women can leverage these differences as strengths to level up in both their personal and professional lives"— Provided by publisher.
Identifiers: LCCN 2020051839 (print) | LCCN 2020051840 (ebook) | ISBN 9780310361206 (hardcover) | ISBN 9780310361213 (ebook)
Subjects: LCSH: Thought and thinking. | Women—Research. | Brain—Research.
Classification: LCC BF441 .A44 2021 (print) | LCC BF441 (ebook) | DDC 153.4/2—dc23
LC record available at https://lccn.loc.gov/2020051839
LC ebook record available at https://lccn.loc.gov/2020051840

Published in association with The Bindery Agency, www.TheBinderyAgency.com.

Zondervan Thrive, an imprint of Zondervan, publishes books that empower readers with insightful, expert-driven ideas for a life of thriving in today's world.

Cover design: Curt Diepenhorst
Cover illustration: Mario Pantelic / Shutterstock
Interior design: Mallory Collins

Printed in the United States of America

---

21 22 23 24 25   /LSC/   10 9 8 7 6 5 4 3 2 1

To Rita, my grandmother, whose indomitable spirit and sense of adventure were ahead of her time and left a blueprint for me. I hope you are looking down proudly. Love you.

Contents

Contents

Preface

To many, an exclamation point is nothing more than a punctuation mark. But to Nancy Camarota it was odd, very odd. She leaned over her desk to stare at the email. She didn't know she was the recipient of consulting company Deloitte's new strategy to approach women differently than men or that this strategy was the brainchild of Cathy Benko, vice chairman and managing principal at Deloitte. Benko encourages her team "to understand where women are coming from"[1] because businesswomen shop for services differently than men.

Benko learned this the hard way. Just two years earlier, her team lost out on a multimillion-dollar account with a hospital. At first, they were mystified. What had they done wrong? They had spent hours going over their pitch, taking care to adopt the perspective of their potential client. During the presentation, the team felt confident that they had covered all the issues raised. But Bill Pelster, one of the senior partners on Benko's team, later described that the rapport felt "off," that the team and client representatives were never on the same wavelength. It was only later that Pelster realized why: half the hospital reps were women.

In a high stakes meeting like that, the team should have significantly altered their pitch to match their audience.

Since then, Benko has been championing a shift to adapt to women in the workplace, from punctuation in emails, to seating arrangements during negotiations, to purchasing behavior. It came as a surprise to Benko to discover that at the time, analysts did relatively little research on the purchasing behavior of women. So Pelster and Benko decided to undertake some research of their own. They interviewed men and women from eighteen large organizations and used their insights to create a playbook to understand female decision-making in the workplace.[2]

Benko was a trailblazer. She realized that not enough was being done to cater to a growing market, and it was bad for business. She also saw that very little research on how women think and approach problem-solving had left the ivory tower of academia and made its way to the public.

This book addresses that gap. This isn't a book about how women are better than men or how the world got it wrong about us. It is a book I wish I had read when I was finding my way into adulthood. This book looks at the statements we hear, the myths we tell ourselves, the platitudes we recite—and pulls back the curtain to see what is really happening inside a woman's head.

While substantial evidence reveals that our brains are structurally different from men's, it is far from deterministic. This is not an attempt to compartmentalize men and women. We operate on a spectrum, and it is better to classify behaviors as adaptive versus maladaptive, rather than good or bad. After all, as we will see throughout this book, context can turn one "good" behavior into a "bad" one.

Women's brains are different. Thanks to a growing body of

scientific research, we know how these differences develop across the lifespan. Despite the tremendous growth in our knowledge and understanding about the brain, in many ways we still adopt a one-size-fits-both (men and women) approach when it comes to everyday behaviors. Glance at any research study and you will quickly see that the results are seldom parsed out by how the females differed from the males.

Why does that matter? It matters because, as women, we often underestimate our abilities, downplay our successes, or apologize for asking questions. At a recent conference, when I complimented a presenter on her talk, she quickly responded, "It was nothing. You should hear some of my other colleagues' work!" This type of response is common. A study done at Cornell University reported that women underestimate both their abilities and their performance, in contrast to men, who overestimate both. However, the researchers found that the women did not *actually* differ in the quality or quantity of their performance from men.[3]

As women, we suffer from "imposter syndrome," wondering, "Are we really good enough?" The data bears this out: a report by a Fortune 500 company disclosed that men apply for a job even if they meet only 60 percent of the qualifications. But women won't apply unless they feel 100 percent qualified![4]

As a woman and a psychologist, I have grown increasingly interested in this disconnect between our abilities and our behavior. I've spent my career researching and sharing landmark findings in working memory, a field of brain science that didn't receive a lot of attention previously. This critical brain process is the ability to hold information in mind for a brief period and do something with that data while ignoring any distractions.

Through my research, I realized that the female brain processes information differently in key ways, so I shifted the focus of my research and consulting to the female brain. The more I delved into this fascinating area, the more I was able to zero in on ways women can benefit from this knowledge and harness it for their own advantage.

On the speaker circuit, I share my insights about the brain with Fortune 500 companies, including Prudential, World Bank, Holland & Knight, and Black Knight. In the past few years, a growing number of corporations and women's organizations, such as chapters of the National Association of Women Business Owners (the voice of more than 10 million women-owned businesses in the US), have asked me to educate them about the female brain and how we can all harness its power. I've emerged as a media-friendly spokesperson for the power of brain processing, explaining how women can take advantage of their unique neural traits to excel daily in every aspect of their lives. You may have seen me on *Good Morning America*, caught my TEDx Talk, or seen me on any of dozens of other media appearances. You may have read about my research in the *New York Times*, the *Wall Street Journal*, *Forbes*, or *Bloomberg* or read one of my seven books (six academic books and one trade book, *The Working Memory Advantage*, Simon & Schuster, 2013). You can catch episodes of a new ABC/NBC series launched in May 2018 called *This Is Me*, in which the hosts explore my expertise to discover how women can engage in everyday activities to maximize their working memory, boost their cognitive and decision-making skills, and solidify competence at work. I'm also under consideration for a Travel Channel pilot in which I would provide expert commentary on what's happening in the brain during a variety of emotional experiences, such as when you're faced with stress or anxiety at work. And in my psychology practice, I help many women learn how to use their uniquely female brain to live their best lives.

So let me share with you the ten ways in which women can boss up, step up, and realize what the brain is capable of doing.

Acknowledgments

On the first day of school, my teacher sent home the report that "Tracy is a social butterfly and spent the day going from desk to desk, making sure that everyone was happy." Fast-forward a few (!) years, and not much has changed. I still love flitting from conversation to conversation and learning new things from each exchange.

My predilection for socializing meant that writing this book during the pandemic when social distancing was in place was especially hard. This has made me especially grateful for the cheerleaders in my life. Some I have not actually met in person, like connections on social media who have messaged me encouragements, shared their perspective, and participated in the polls that I talk about in this book.

I am also grateful for friends who have taken me to coffee and early morning paddleboarding sessions where I could bounce ideas off them as they germinated. Thanks to friends who read my chapters as they were still forming and I felt so nervous about sharing them. And thanks to those who were always on the other end of the phone to make me laugh whenever I hit a wall. These many wonderful people buoyed me up when I needed it most.

Acknowledgments

The women in this book are truly an inspiration to me: Christine Hoene, Eden Kendall, Chloe Hakim-Moore, and Elena Gomez. Thank you for setting the bar high and for letting me share your stories.

Thank you to my agent, Alexander Field, for helping me breathe life into my vision. From our very first email, I felt that you really understood what I wanted to share with this book. I hit the jackpot with the team at Zondervan Books/HarperCollins. Stephanie Smith, my editor, has been so encouraging and supportive. She exudes this light and breeziness that made me feel that whatever writer's block I had was entirely surmountable. Thanks to Kim Tanner for the editorial direction that gently nudged me back to the surface when I would get bogged down. And thank you, Bridgette Brooks and Trinity McFadden, whose marketing eye has been instrumental in creating a look that matches what I want to share in this book.

My family has been a bastion of support, from countless discussions, to reading (very rough!) drafts, to sharing my excitement about each stage of the process. Thank you for believing in me.

Part One

The Decision-Making Brain

One

The Stressed Brain

Strategies for Women to Make
Sound Decisions under Stress

"Code violation. Racket abuse. Point penalty, Mrs. Williams."
The ESPN camera zoomed in to a tight shot of the broken frame
of her tennis racket lying on the court. It was the 2018 US Open
women's final, and Serena Williams was one win short of tying
the record for twenty-four Grand Slam singles titles.

But it wasn't going well.

This was her second penalty point. The first was a controversial code violation for receiving coaching when the umpire
said he witnessed William's coach giving her a thumbs up. In
response to the umpire's second call, Williams demanded that
he apologize, as he had "attacked [her] character" and "insinu-
ated that [she] was cheating." She put her towel down and looked
directly at the umpire. "You stole a point from me. You're a thief

3

too."[1] She got up and walked away. "Code violation. Verbal abuse. Game penalty, Mrs. Williams."[2] Game. Set. Match.

Serena Williams's response has fueled heated debate, drawing both support and criticism for her actions. Williams had the support of the twenty thousand–strong crowd, who responded to the umpire's call with jeers and boos. But she also drew sharp criticism. Some likened her response to a "temper tantrum like a four-year-old,"[3] feeding the misperception that women are more emotional under stress and make poor decisions as a result.

Tennis legend Billie Jean King, who has won thirty-nine Grand Slam titles (twelve singles and the rest in doubles) captured the sentiment when she said, "When a woman is emotional, she's 'hysterical' and she's penalized for it. When a man does the same, he's 'outspoken' and there are no repercussions." King is not wrong. When Andy Murray, winner of three Grand Slam titles, kicked a ball toward an umpire's head during the 2016 Cincinnati Masters in Ohio, the media joked that he "showed off his football skills."[4] He received no penalty. Roger Federer, in the 2009 US Open men's final, swore multiple times at the umpire and got off with the equivalent of a slap on the wrist—a small fine. Not a game penalty. Andre Agassi similarly insulted the umpire at the US Open in 1990 and even spat on him. His penalty? A fine issued five days *after* the match.

Footage of Williams talking to the umpire after receiving the first point penalty shows her as calm and even respectful. In subsequent interviews, she defended her behavior, saying that the umpire "has never taken a game from a man because they said 'thief.'"[5] Her motivations behind her behavior appear to be driven for a desire to have a single standard for male and female players. "I just feel like the fact that I have to go through this is just an example for the next person that has emotions, and that wants to express themselves, and want to be a strong woman. They're going to be allowed to do that because of today."[6]

While there is certainly a social double standard about the emotional response to a stressful situation in sports, what does science have to say about how stress affects men and women when it comes to decision-making?

Myth:

Women make emotional decisions when they are stressed.

Psychologists talk about two brain pathways involved in decision-making: an emotional path, governed by the amygdala, and a rational one, governed by the prefrontal cortex. The amygdala is involved when faced with difficult decisions that have emotional implications. Neurobiology professor Larry Cahill edited an entire neuroscience journal dedicated to understanding how brain functions affect men and women differently.[7] For starters, a man's amygdala is larger than a woman's. It also works differently. Psychologists report that while both men and women are concerned about the outcome of their decisions, especially in moral dilemmas, women care much more about avoiding harm. This means we are more likely to avoid "rational" decisions in favor of more "emotional" ones. So we might conclude that the stereotype is true in some situations. But we can flip the switch and override the emotional decision-making default.

The Runaway Trolley

Alison shifted uncomfortably. "I can't choose. I just can't. It's too hard." She pushed her back up against the chair and pulled nervously at the Velcro straps attached to her fingers. "Can I skip this one?"

Alison was sitting in my research lab, facing a computer screen. On it was displayed a familiar scenario, one that philosophers have been using for decades to explore moral decision-making. The setup is simple: Would you kill one person to save five? You see a runaway trolley car hurtling down the tracks, and if you pull a lever, you can switch the tracks, saving the five people who are standing unsuspectingly in its path. The catch, and there's always a catch in these thought experiments, is that switching tracks means you are responsible for the death of one person standing on track two.

The equipment I was using measured Alison's physiological response to stress. Sometimes called the "truth maker" because it reveals what your words try to mask, this equipment measures what your body does when it encounters an arousing stimulus. Arousal leads to an increase of adrenaline, which leads to tiny beads of sweat. This is what I was measuring using metal cuffs held on to Alison's fingers with Velcro. The interesting thing about this equipment is that it couldn't tell me whether Alison was happy, sad, or afraid. It showed me only how *intense* her emotions were. Right now, her emotions were heightened.

Lucky for me, more sophisticated equipment has already marked what happens when we encounter these moral scenarios. Joshua Greene, who began his academic journey as a philosopher, found that when women are faced with the dilemma of taking a life, even if it saves five, we don't always adopt a consequentialist approach, meaning that we don't always agree that the end justifies the means. Instead we express a strong emotional reaction, at least in our brains. When he placed people in an fMRI machine, he found that the decision to pull the lever corresponded with activity in the prefrontal cortex, indicating a contemplated and conscious decision. Conversely, in another version of the scenario where the reader was directly involved in the death of the innocent bystander (like pushing someone on the main track), the amygdala, which is the brain's emotional center, was activated.[8]

In an interview with *BrainWorld* in 2019, Greene described the two decision-making pathways as a digital SLR camera: "You've got your automatic settings (emotional brain) and your manual mode (the rational brain). Which way of taking photos is better? Neither is absolutely better. The manual and automatic settings are good for different things. If you're doing something standard, with pretty typical goals in mind, point-and-shoot settings are probably better. But if you're trying to do something fancy, something the manufacturer of the camera didn't envision, then you want to put the camera in manual mode."[9] In everyday moral problems, the automatic setting works—don't lie, don't steal. But with more complex ethical dilemmas, we need the manual setting.

Research shows us that women want to avoid harm against others, so we are more likely to favor an emotional decision. But does this help us make better decisions? Well, that depends. The feeling brain is powerful: it can help you turn the focus away from you and prioritize someone else when you have to make a decision. However, if you are in a position where

Truth:

In many cases, women do naturally use the automatic setting of emotional decisions, but they can also make rational decisions if they know how to flip their brain switch.

you are giving up something you want (for example, a job offer) because you are worried about your decision negatively affecting someone else (like your current boss), then the automatic setting may not be a positive thing. So how can you flip the switch in your brain and make a rational decision? The answer may lie in something unexpected, something you usually try to avoid: stress.

The Trolley Experiment

Alison was one of over one hundred participants who sat in my lab as they listened to different moral dilemmas. But that was not all. During some of these dilemmas, Alison and the other participants were asked to stick their left hand in a bucket of ice water chilled to around 34 degrees Fahrenheit for one minute. This task is designed to elevate stress levels. A chain reaction happens in the brain once it detects a stressor (in this case, icy water is the physical stressor): the hypothalamus in the brain, which is responsible for our stress response, activates part of our autonomic nervous system and releases adrenaline in preparation for a fight-or-flight response.

Just for fun, I added another stressor. This time, a cognitive stressor. I asked Alison and the others to count backward by sixes, starting from one hundred, while listening to the moral dilemmas. Researchers have reported that mental arithmetic tasks like this one also elevate stress levels. This pattern held true in my study. Alison and the other participants reported feeling more stressed when counting backward as quickly and accurately as possible. The metal cuffs on their fingers provided further evidence: they were significantly sweatier than when they were not counting.

Both the physical and cognitive stressors can change a woman's default decision-making strategies. Both the physical stressor (ice water) and the cognitive stressor (counting backward) flipped a switch in their brains. And they changed their initial emotional response to a more rational one. Now when presented with the trolley dilemma, the women didn't shy away from saving the five people. Instead, they were more likely to sacrifice one person for the greater good.

Why? For women, the default mode in tough emotional decisions is to reduce harm, which relies on the amygdala. But with a stressor introduced, the amygdala is occupied, first with sounding the alarm in response to the stressor, then with deactivating after the stressor is removed. This creates a window of opportunity for the prefrontal cortex, the rational part of the brain, to step in and take over. The prefrontal cortex sits in the front of our brain, aptly located, like a ruler taking charge of the rest of our sometimes impulsive and unruly cognitive functions.

Turning On Your Rational Brain

A team of scientists from Italy explored how the prefrontal cortex works when men and women have to choose between rational and emotional decisions.[10] They used a technique called transcranial direct current stimulation. It is a noninvasive technique that uses short magnetic pulses to stimulate specific brain regions. Just like in my study with the stressors, they found a difference in how men and women responded. A shock to the prefrontal cortex changed women's answers to the trolley dilemma, and they were more likely to make a rational decision. But for men, nothing changed.

Why did the magnets flip a switch in the women's brains? When it comes to tough decisions that have moral implications, women focus more on avoiding directly causing harm to someone. They downplay messages from the prefrontal cortex that tell them to focus on decisions that benefit the greater good. The magnetic pulses stimulated the prefrontal cortex, giving it a boost. For women, this small boost was enough to shift their attention when making moral decisions.

Under stress, women make more rational decisions than emotional ones.

If you need to turn down your feeling brain, stress can be a helpful tool. Stress in a short period (just one minute) overloads your feeling brain so you can flip the switch to using your rational brain in decision-making. A physical stressor, like sticking your hand in a bucket of ice water for one minute, can flip off the switch for your feeling brain. While your amygdala is busy focusing on the discomfort from the icy water, your prefrontal cortex has a window of opportunity to explore your options in a rational and objective manner. Adding a cognitive stress, like counting backward from one hundred in sixes (100, 94, 88, 82 . . .), is another way to turn down the volume of your feeling brain and give your rational brain a chance to make a decision.

From Trolleys to Cars

Mary Barra, the first female CEO of General Motors (GM), is no stranger to making decisions under pressure. She was promoted at a time when GM was experiencing one of the worst safety crises in the auto industry. It was under scrutiny for failing to recall vehicles that had a faulty ignition switch. This led to 275 injuries and 124 deaths. Barra acted quickly. She hired independent experts to conduct an internal investigation. She appointed a new vice president of global safety. She oversaw instigated recalls of more than thirty million vehicles. Her efforts paid off. She is widely credited for reaching an agreement with federal regulators in record time.[11]

Barra is considered a GM lifer—she had already spent thirty-three years at the company before her rise to CEO. Efficiency had already characterized her leadership style. For example, as head of human resources five years previously, she truncated ten pages of dress code guidelines to two words: *dress appropriately.* Yet when she took over GM, many saw her promotion not as an indication of her competence and success in the workplace but as an example of the "glass cliff" in practice.

Two British psychologists coined the term "glass cliff" to characterize a phenomenon in the workplace of hiring female executives during a crisis and then ditching them when they can't fix it.[12] But Barra overturned this stereotype. While it is true that she was hired during a time of crisis, GM had burned through five male CEOs in the six years prior to Barra taking the helm. Fast-forward five years after Barra's appointment and she is still successfully leading GM.

In 2018 Barra again made headlines when GM announced the closing of plants that would lead to a loss of fourteen thousand employees. The parallels between this decision and the hypothetical trolley dilemma are interesting. In both cases, sacrifices were made for a greater good: to save five people in the trolley dilemma and to facilitate a culture of economic growth, as Barra sees it. Not everyone sees it this way. GM and Barra have received heat for this decision, both from Congress, who perceives it as a betrayal after government bailouts, and from the workers, who feel that their loyalty to GM was misguided.

Science tells us that the amygdala is involved when faced with difficult decisions that have emotional implications (layoffs of loyal employees for Barra and the hypothetical demise of innocents in the trolley dilemma). Remember that women typically want to avoid harm, so they are more likely to favor an emotional decision.

But that is not what Barra did. On the surface, it seems that the decision to close plants directly results in harm because of the layoffs of thousands of GM employees. Barra made a rational decision, one that results in a greater good: the growth of the company.

From Ice to Magnets

So why were Barra's actions counter to what science predicted? Because of stress. Barra didn't ignore her feeling brain. When dealing with the safety crisis, she made the decision to meet with families of the accident victims. "I put myself in their shoes and thought they deserved to be heard," Barra said.[13] And she wasn't about lip service. She spent hours listening and apologizing as she heard families share their loss. She was clearly moved, and there are reports of her holding back tears as she met them. But she didn't need a zap to the prefrontal cortex to make a considered and rational decision that resulted in the greater good. All it took was a little bit of stress.

If you find yourself in a position of needing to make a rational decision, but feel pulled emotionally, perhaps a bucket of ice water could be your new best friend.

Summary: Women make emotional decisions from a desire to avoid harming someone. But under stress, women often make rational decisions.

Think Like a Girl

Use stress to flip the switch from your emotional brain to your rational brain in decision-making.

1. **Chill!**

   Try adding a physical stressor, such as sticking your hand in a bucket of ice water for one minute.
2. **Count.**

   Add a cognitive stress, such as counting backward from one hundred by sixes (100, 94, 88, 82 . . .) or by threes (100, 97, 94, 91 . . .).

Two

The Risk-Taking Brain

How Women Uniquely Evaluate Risk

Aroo!

Eden holds up her thumb to me. "See, I cut myself on barbed wire!" We are sitting in comfy chairs at the CW TV studio. Eden is a Spartan. Not just any Spartan. A Spartan who has made it to the podium multiple times (that is, won a medal in her age group) at national competitions, including the Beast. The Beast is a grueling half marathon filled with almost impossible obstacles, such as climbing up slippery walls pitched at an inverted angle, crawling under barbed wire, and jumping over fire, that "will challenge everything you're made of,"[1] according to the Spartan website. Spartan races are now in more than forty countries on six continents and have garnered a somewhat cultlike following among fitness enthusiasts.

As with any community, Spartans have their own ways of

inspiring each other, including training programs, family events in the form of Spartan Kids races, and even their own chant: *Aroo!* As one race ambassador wrote on Reddit, "We use **AROO** to express positive excitement or in agreement with a person."

As a TV host, Eden shares that she frequently gets comments about her training-induced bruising. "Why would you want to have your legs look like that?" and "Don't you realize you are on TV?" She pauses and grins at me. "Why do I do it? Because it is so much fun! It's an adventure. I want to try new things!" I have had the privilege of working with Eden for several years as a frequent guest on the *Morning Show.* Now she is trying to persuade me to join her on a Spartan race. Her mangled thumb is not helping her case. But is the Spartan race so different from some of my childhood activities?

I was that girl with the purple knees. Growing up in Malaysia meant a lot of outdoor time. Television programming didn't start till later in the day, and besides, we weren't allowed screen time during the week. Luckily the neighborhood we lived in was tree-lined and had a park close by. Monkey bars were my favorite, and I would happily spend afternoons swinging from bar to bar. Of course, I took an occasional fall, and my mom would be quick to dab iodine on my knees. The bright purple color from the iodine was a reminder of the risk that even fun activities carry. Of course, that didn't deter me from heading back out the next day.

Would you play on monkey bars today? As adults, we seem to lose some of our childhood courage. Activities that we found fun and exciting as kids now seem dangerous and risky.

Eden tells me about the monkey bars in the Spartan race. These aren't your average playground monkey bars. These Spartan monkey bars spin and swivel every time you reach out to grip them. Set eight feet above the ground, they also increase and decrease in height. To make it even more challenging, the bars are about two feet apart from each other, so if you aren't blessed with a Michael Phelps–like arm span, you have to take a wild leap and hope you don't fall. Oh, and there is no safety net.

Myth:

Women take fewer risks than men.

Abundant research reveals that women are less prone to *physical* risk-taking than men. Yet Eden doesn't view activities like the Spartan races as risky. "I train hard. Every time I see a new obstacle, I think, 'I don't think I can do this obstacle.' Baby steps, and I get there. I plan it. I know what to expect."[2] "Is Eden an anomaly?" I wondered.

As I looked into the stats on risk-taking, I saw that some of the results may be skewed. Typically, research questions on risk-taking have been biased toward "male" activities. But when British researchers included new activities that diverged from "conventional macho measures of daring, such as betting vast sums on a football game," they found that women rated themselves as equally or more likely to take risks.[3]

How Much Risk Is Too Much?

Before we go much further into how women make decisions about taking risks, what is risk? Professor James Byrnes and his colleagues at the University of Maryland defined risk-taking behavior in part by the negative consequences of that behavior (like basically all the *Jackass* stunts).[4]

So how does an obstacle course race stack up? Let's start by defining "negative consequences" as the percentage of injuries.

Obstacle course races are typically held outdoors, where some obstacles involve swimming and holding your breath in "unfriendly" terrains, like icy lakes and swamp water. It's not hard to imagine that the risk of injury is quadruple what it would be on a pleasant run in your neighborhood. One doctor is reported as saying, "Winning is not the goal. Crossing the finish line standing upright is the goal."[5]

Reports from obstacle-race competitors fuel the notion of it being a high-risk activity. Reports of infections from swallowing muddy water, to sticks piercing through a foot, to hypothermia abound. It's not only the obstacles that bring out the sense of competition. Injuries seem to be equally competitive, with athletes trying to one-up each other for the best bragging rights. But the actual injury count is less sensational than the stories. A study that looked at onsite reports of injuries at thirty-three obstacle course racing events from over seventy thousand competitors found that only 2.4 percent had injuries. And of these injuries, only 1 percent of them required emergency medical services. This included fractures, dehydration (only one competitor), and heat stroke (also only one competitor). The majority of the injuries were cuts, scrapes, strains, and sprains and were treatable on site.[6]

Here's the thing about risk: You don't make decisions based on the number of actual injuries. You make decisions based on the *perception* of risk. Consider the actual number of injuries from a common physical activity: running. According to the Harvard Medical School, anywhere from 30 to 75 percent of runners are injured annually, with repetitive stress injuries being the biggest complaint.[7] Yet the majority of us perceive running as far less risky than completing an obstacle course race. Of course if someone were to run multiple obstacle races in a year, the percentages might be closer, but the idea is that the perceived risk of running an obstacle race is higher than the actual risk.

Actual Risk versus Perceived Risk

Reported injuries are one way to measure the risk of participating in certain activities. There is a more macabre calculation: the likelihood of sudden death. A micromort does this. It is a unit of risk of an activity. One micromort is a one-in-a-million chance of death. A healthy activity like running a marathon is 7 micromorts per run, which is pretty close to skydiving, at 10 micromorts per jump.[8] While this number sounds small, compare this with the risk of driving a car for 333 miles a mere 1 in a million chance of dying!

To take a closer look at how we perceive risk, I took to social media to gain a real-world understanding of this topic. I asked my twenty-five thousand Instagram followers to decide which of two options was less risky. Here's how the responses stacked up and how they compare with the actual risk calculation using micromorts.

	Running	vs.	Skydiving
Percent of people who see it as riskier	32%		68%
Micromorts (actual risk)	7 micromorts per run		10 micromorts per jump

	Swimming	vs.	Driving a car 333 miles
Responses	22%		78%
Micromorts (actual risk)	12 micromorts (chance of drowning)		1 micromort

	Biking for 28 miles	vs.	Skiing
Responses	24%		76%
Micromorts (actual risk)	1 micromort		< 1 micromort per day

The responses from my poll are clear: we are poor judges of what activities are *actually* risky. Every day, you may participate in relatively high-risk activities like running, swimming, and bike riding, in part because you perceive them to be low risk. (To be sure, abundant evidence reveals that these activities offer substantial cardiovascular and even mental health benefits. But in this conversation, we are talking about the perception of risk versus actual risk.)

How Many Micromorts in a Selfie

Many of us participate in activities with higher actual risk because we don't perceive them as risky. Consider, for example, a ubiquitous activity that anyone can do. It requires no skill and little preparation: taking selfies. This activity seems innocuous enough, but a study in the *Journal of Family Medicine and Primary Care* calculated that from October 2011 to November 2017, 259 people died while taking a selfie, rising sharply from just three reported selfie-related deaths in 2011 to ninety-three selfie-related deaths in 2017.[9]

Risk theory assumes that we are rational beings and that we will review possible outcomes and weigh the severity of the consequences of our actions. It presupposes that we have an in-built decision-making metric that cleverly guides us to make informed and safe decisions. But these cognitive theories can't explain why some of us don't calculate the risk of standing at the edge of a cliff or floating in radioactive waters just to take a selfie, ignoring reports of rashes that appear after being at these picturesque but toxic locations. Such risky behavior is widespread too: in my

Instagram poll, 74 percent of people said they would take a "risky selfie."

If we aren't good at assessing actual risk, then what do we use to determine the perception of risk? Carnegie Mellon researchers Lowenstein and colleagues suggest a different theory to explain risky behavior. We use our *feelings* to judge the risk level of an activity. If you *like* an activity, you judge the risks as low and the benefits as high. If you *dislike* an activity, you do the opposite: you view the activity as high risk with low benefits. They call this "risk as feelings."[10]

Selfie-taking captures this sentiment of how feelings direct risk-taking behavior. Selfies make you feel good. When a group of researchers from the University of California asked people to take selfies of themselves every day for four weeks, they found that smiling selfies made them feel happy. When *Euronews* interviewed me on the topic of risky selfies, I shared that when we see a "like" or a positive comment on our feed or post, there's a huge dopamine rush, and that's a feel-good hormone. Dopamine also helps to reinforce a certain behavior, so if a picture gets a lot of likes or positive attention, that encourages us to post another selfie. Social media can offer enjoyment and pleasure. As a result, you think of standing at the edge of a cliff to take a selfie as low risk and consider social validation from that photo as a high benefit.

Risk-Taking as Emotions

Women are thought to have high levels of *emotional responsiveness*. Researchers suggest that this pattern translates to us experiencing emotions more intensely than men. Does this affect our risk-taking? Psychologist Christine Harris and her colleagues from the University of San Diego took a closer look at this question in relation to extreme sports such as:

- going whitewater rafting during rapid water flows in the spring
- periodically engaging in a dangerous sport (for example, mountain climbing or skydiving)
- piloting your own small plane, if you could
- chasing a tornado or hurricane by car to take dramatic photos

Over six hundred adults responded to her questions about how they felt about these activities. As with many other studies on risk-taking, women felt that these activities would likely end badly for them. But Harris found an interesting twist.

Feelings matter, especially to women. They mattered so much that they determined whether the women would participate in these risky activities. The same pattern was not true for the male participants. Compare Harris's data on extreme sports with my risky-selfie poll: Over two-thirds of women said they would take a risky selfie! If women enjoy an activity, they are more likely to take that risk.

Remember Eden from the beginning of the chapter? She understood the power of emotions in decision-making and was willing to trade the fear of the unknown in the moment for the reward in the future. The dopamine hit she gets from a Spartan race is clearly a motivating factor. "Doing a Spartan race is like a reward. Every time I overcame something, I would get more excited."[11]

When you are faced with making a risky decision, listen to

your emotions to judge the risk level of an activity, while recognizing that your like or dislike of it will influence your feelings about it. This will help you determine some objectivity about the risk ahead of you. And your emotions can also help you recognize an immediate fear or concern and whether there is a greater emotional payoff to come.

Risk versus Return

I am not a risk taker. That is what I told myself as I peered out from the gaping hole in the plane as it soared 12,500 feet above the ground. I tugged at the straps that hugged my chest. "Any pro tips?" I asked. "Don't look down," my tandem instructor replied without even breaking into a smile. He nudged me toward the hole where the door should have been. I told myself, "Look up! Look up! Look u—" Then I felt nothing beneath my feet. The wind sounded so loud that even if I screamed, no one would hear. And then there was silence. Absolute silence. No voices, no ambient noise. It was the most peaceful feeling I have ever experienced. At this point, I should confess something: I have a fear of heights. I sometimes close my eyes when I walk across a bridge. So you may wonder why I willingly chose to jump out of a plane.

When women evaluate risk, we use a calculation—not one based on probabilities of different outcomes but one that brings emotions to the center. The calculation looks at a trade-off between what you get from the choice based on what you invest. Harris's data is one of the first pieces of research to substantiate this link. She created a list

Truth:

Women do pursue risks.

of scenarios that had high potential payoffs and relatively minor but certain costs:

- trying to sell a screenplay, which you have already written, to a Hollywood film studio
- calling a radio station where the twelfth caller will win a month's worth of income
- sending out thirty applications for high-paying jobs after graduating from college
- regularly visiting a professor in her office hours and then asking her for a letter of recommendation

Now the tables were turned. Harris found that women reported more positive consequences from these scenarios, which led to women being more likely than men to participate in them.[12] This pattern was opposite of the vast majority of studies on risk-taking where women take fewer risks than men. In a meta-analysis where researchers reviewed over 150 papers on risk perception, this pattern that women take fewer risks was true across self-reported activities, like smoking and driving, as well as observed behavior involving physical activity.[13] Even in the accidents from the selfie-taking study described previously, less than a quarter of the victims were women.

Why did Harris find such a different pattern? A compelling reason is that research has primarily focused on a consequentialist approach: that you make decisions based on your assessments of the probability of certain consequences. But that approach ignores the fact that women use a different metric. We are aware of the consequences, and we judge them to be highly valuable. Researchers call this the *risk-return framework*. Emotions play a big role. A woman would be willing to trade fear in the present for positive emotion in the future and take a greater risk in one activity if she gets her expected returns.

Our risk calculations are different from men's, but we're willing to take just as many risks—as long as we see the potential for a return. This approach does involve some longer-term thinking because you have to overlook discomfort now for happiness later. If you recognize how your brain sees the risk, then you can be more confident taking risks.

As I floated through the air, I had made a calculation too. I was willing to trade my fear of heights for the incredible exhilaration of flying for the first time.

This risk calculation can be a therapeutic outlet, as I discovered when I interviewed Spartan race director Garfield Griffiths as part of the *Morning Show* with Eden. He shared that some people come to do a Spartan race to get away from stress or something negative in their life, saying, "It's very hard to think about anything else that's going on when you have to climb an eight-foot wall and you have to go through a swamp under barbed wire."[14]

One group of women especially benefits from the Spartan races. Rethreaded is a business that employs survivors of human trafficking. For the last three years, the women at Rethreaded have participated in the Spartan races. For Janene, one obstacle filled her with dread and tempted her to give up: the inverted incline wall, which is set at a 70-degree reverse angle. But she did it. Janene and others from the Rethreaded community have similar experiences, and their stories speak volumes of how they are willing to trade fear in the moment for that sense of accomplishment at the end. "I didn't know how strong I was. I didn't know that was possible. I'm so glad that I did it."[15] They take the risk because the reward of seeing how strong they are builds their confidence.

For Eden, and thousands of other Spartan competitors, the decision to sign up for an obstacle course race is not a cognitive decision; it is an emotional one. And it is a decision that is worth the initial fear.

Summary: Women do pursue risks; we use a different calculation to evaluate risk—not one based on probabilities of different outcomes but one that brings emotions to the center. It is a calculation that looks at a trade-off between what you get from it based on what you invest.

Think Like a Girl

When you are faced with making a risky decision, listen to your emotions.

1. **Feel your decision.**

   Pay attention to your *feelings* to judge the risk level of an activity. If you like an activity, you judge the risks as low and the benefits as high. If you dislike an activity, you do the opposite: you view the activity as high risk with low benefits.

2. **Consider what you will get in return.**

   You are likely to take a greater risk in one activity if you get your expected returns. Think beyond the moment to the long-term. What discomfort will you need to overlook now? And what will be the happiness or reward in the future? If the future payoff is greater than the current discomfort, take your risk confidently.

Part Two

The Love Brain

Three

The Romantic Brain

What Women Should Really Look for in a Partner

The English language has only one word for *love*. We use that same word to describe the feeling we have for our partners, our parents, and our children. But consider Sanskrit, a language that has influenced many Asian languages. Sanskrit has almost one hundred words for love, ranging from maternal love to passionate love to a term that is sometimes used as a name for young girls (roughly translated to "darling"). It's not only classical languages that have multiple words for love; Arabic and Irish do too. While the language we use to describe love appears to be culturally specific, the emotions are not. It appears that the feelings associated with love are universal, according to researchers who studied more than 166 societies, including the Mediterranean, Africa, the Americas, Asia, and the Pacific islands. They first started their search by looking at ethnographic accounts of these cultures.

Next they scoured love songs, folklores, and native accounts of romantic love. Romantic love, according to the researchers, was an "intense attraction that involves the idealization of the other."[1] It would typically lead to an immediate commitment that may be short-term. This characterization of romantic love relates to the *attraction stage*, rather than the *attachment phase*, where individuals experience growth and satisfaction in their relationship.

The researchers argue that documented instances of romantic love in cultures around the world are strong evidence that love is a universal feeling and not just a Western idea. We all experience the rush of attraction and desire to pursue it. Evidence of romantic love was reported in almost 90 percent of the societies they explored. For example, a woman living in a desert society is recorded as saying that her relationship with her husband is "rich, warm and secure" and that "when two people come together their hearts are on fire and their passion is very great."[2]

The angst of love beyond reach and the yearning to grasp it has universal echoes. A folklore from the Song dynasty era (AD 960–1279) talks about a young man who falls in love with a woman who is already betrothed to another man. This young man felt that "the greatest desire of his was beyond him."[3] In his despair, he loses interest in his daily activities. Then one day he decides to summon the courage to confess his feelings of love to the young woman and learns that she has similar feelings for him. They run away together, but hardship and poverty befall them. As they contemplate leaving each other to return to their former lives, the young man looks deeply into his lover's eyes and says, "Since heaven and earth were created, you were made for me and I will not let you go. It cannot be wrong to love you."[4]

"A grown-up love story should not be a fairy tale or a romantic tragedy, but instead should be approached as a mystery," suggests professor Ty Tashiro at the University of Maryland.[5] Yet perhaps the biggest mystery is why we fall in love with the people that we do. How many times have you seen the person your friend is dating and thought they seemed like an odd match? Not only would you not date them, but you are also surprised that your friend can't stop talking about their new partner.

What do you think love is? Let's first explore love as attraction. Attraction relates to the first phase of love: the excitement, that giddy rush, and the inexplicable urge to spend all your time with someone (the chemicals are real!). In the next chapter, we'll explore love as attachment: the warm, comfortable, dependable nature of love (the feeling that you could spend all day in your PJs together and still have a good time with the one you love).

Attraction: Love Rewards in the Beginning

Close your eyes. Think of a fun event you recently shared with a love interest or partner. Did you know that this simple action brings a rush of reward to your brain? Dopamine is a feel-good hormone that is released by a myriad of activities, including a delicious meal, a good conversation, and even when you get a like on your social media post.

Romantic love is like a reward in our brain circuitry. It happens in the caudate nucleus and ventral tegmental area, both of which are the reward centers of the brain. Researchers have found that it happens in the early stages of intense romantic love. Some scientists have likened the sensation of early love to cocaine addiction in animals. It creates the same sense of euphoria, boundless energy, restlessness, and even loss of appetite.

The second thing that happens is that romantic love engages your motivation system. Romantic love targets our secondary reward network. This refers to a reward that in and of itself is not rewarding, but instead, it leads to a reward. Think of money. It is just paper, yet it is more meaningful than monopoly money, which is also paper, because of what it offers: the ability to buy things—and not only tiny plastic houses on a game board.

When you get that hit of dopamine from the rush of the early stages of love, it motivates you to win over that person. You start setting goals and thinking about ways to spend more time with them, conversation topics that would interest them, activities that would make them fall a little bit more in love with you. You move beyond just desiring them to wanting to create a long-term bond with them. The dopamine hit to this secondary reward system means you want to pursue behaviors that psychologists describe as *maintenance* (doing things to make the partner happy) and *protection* (ways to keep your bond with your partner safe and exclusive to you). This powerful combination of reward and motivation has led some psychologists to call love a drive, not a feeling.

Psychologist Arthur Aron recruited people in their early twenties who reported being in love for seven months.[6] Before going into the brain scanner, they indicated how passionately in love they felt, using statements like these:

- I want my partner physically, emotionally, and mentally.
- Sometimes I can't control my thoughts; they are obsessively on my partner.

When the people in Aron's study were lying on their backs in the scanner, they looked at a happy photo they had brought in of their partner. Then they were asked to think about a fun event (not sexual) with their partner as they looked at the photo for thirty seconds. For example:

- "I thought about the time we both woke up at 3 a.m. and walked back from the 7-Eleven store. It was fun walking back and kissing."
- "I felt I could really rely on her; I could open up to her; I felt protected by her."[7]

When they were in the scanner thinking about an event with their partner, they received a huge dopamine shot, which translates into the gushy, giddy, happy feeling called love. And it came just from looking and thinking about their partner for thirty seconds.

The good news is that dopamine sticks around. Researchers looked at men and women who had been in a monogamous relationship for two years who reported being "truly, deeply, and madly in love."[8] The usual reward centers of the brain lit up, showing signs of dopamine at work, producing that feel-good sensation.

If you focus on the happy and fun activities you share with your love, you'll give your brain a reward. But before you spend too much time boosting dopamine via a relationship, you may want to understand what attracted you in the first place and how to make it go the distance. Because the "mystery" of attraction is different for men and women.

The Beginning of Attraction

Myth:

Women should seek out financially stable romantic partners.

Choosing a mate is a big decision. Barry was very cute. So that was definitely a pro. But he knew it too. Hmm, a potential con. Nobody likes a conceited person. So my seven-year-old self was approaching this challenge fully prepared.

I turned to lists. I am a list maker. Maybe this is something I got from my mother. Who knows? Regardless, in big decisions and small ones, I find making lists to be very comforting. In this case, I hoped it would also be insightful.

Pros

- cute
- brown hair
- good smile

Cons

- lots of other girls like him too

Over the years, I kept making lists—when I was faced with job decisions, when to have children, and of course, choosing a partner. Looking back, I wish I knew a lot more of the science behind how to choose a partner as I made my lists.

What are you looking for in a partner? What attracts you in the first place? Are you looking for someone tall, short, brainy, or adventurous? In today's dating world, there is something for everyone. Dating sites range from location-driven, to activity-orientated based on your Facebook connections, to highly specific interests like Sea Captain Date (with the slogan "In the unforgiving ocean of love, let us be your lighthouse"[9]) and Hot Sauce Passions for those who . . . well, you can guess!

Despite this buffet-style approach to catering to our romantic interests, there appears to be a universality in what we are *actually* looking for. David Buss, a psychologist based at the University of Texas, conducted the most comprehensive study exploring the question of what we look for in a partner. He had a sample of over ten thousand people (53 percent female) from thirty-three countries and thirty-seven cultures. While similarities exist across cultures in what we look for in a mate, there are differences between men and women.

You may think that in today's world where women are financially independent, we no longer default to looking for a partner with cash to spare. Yet Buss found that that isn't the case. As a woman, you will likely prefer a partner who is financially secure and has high status. Why do women have this preference? Some researchers suggest that this choice is embedded in our evolutionary history. Women traditionally needed a mate who had sufficient resources to be able to protect them and provide for the family. The same preference occurs in a number of countries.

But ladies, here's the thing about looking for financial stability in a mate: it is a sliding scale with diminishing returns when it comes to happiness in relationships. For couples on the lower end of the income scale, financial stability does contribute to relationship satisfaction. But when your household income is $75,000 a year or higher, financial stability is no longer a big factor in your relationship happiness. This held true in both egalitarian countries, like Sweden and Norway, as well as in less egalitarian cultures, such as Iran. Depending on your income, you may be drawn to financial stability in a mate, but there's more to consider when it comes to happiness and longevity in your relationship.

In contrast, men favor partners who are physically attractive. This is no surprise. Researchers have recently discovered that men already have a pretty good wingman: their brain. Their brain has a special laser that focuses on attractive faces.

Why does this happen? Morphine activates the reward system in the brain. Men see an attractive female face and their brain gets that reward feeling, which makes them want to see more faces. Physical attraction is not just shallow. It has a long-term benefit. According to the researchers, attractiveness is a signal of a mate who has an "evolutionary fitness,"[10] which means they are able to survive in their environment, as well as reproduce. The benefit of the brain's laser focus on attractiveness is that it helps men select a partner who will be able not only to last in a relationship but make the family line last as well. In this case, the brain is in charge, and it dictates what attracts men to a partner.

In today's world, if a woman is financially independent, she may not need a partner for financial reasons. What does science tell us that we should look for in a partner?

Attraction Counts (But Not If You Are a Woman Looking for an Attractive Husband)

What happens when a woman chooses attractiveness? It may not be the right move if you are looking for something long-term.

Attractiveness gets you going in the direction of love, but it doesn't maintain it, as researchers from the University of Tennessee discovered. They recruited eighty-two heterosexual couples in their midtwenties who were within the first six months of their first marriage. Marital satisfaction was measured with questions like the ones listed here:

Truth:

Choosing the right personality type can lead to relationship satisfaction.

How would you respond to these statements about your current romantic relationship?
- We have a good relationship.
- My relationship with my partner makes me happy.
- I feel like part of a team with my partner.
- My relationship with my partner is stable.

The couples were asked to identify a personal problem, or something about themselves they wanted to change. Then they had to talk about it with their partner for ten minutes. The couples were videotaped as they interacted with each other. This served two purposes. The first purpose of the videotaped session was to look at how spouses interact with each other. The researchers looked at things like taking turns in conversation, not talking over their spouse, and overall positivity in their interactions.

The second purpose was to rate the physical attractiveness of each spouse on a scale of 1 to 10 (the higher the rating, the more attractive they were). Several trained research assistants conducted the ratings without knowing how the other researchers were rating the couples (to avoid bias in their perception of attractiveness). While the saying goes that beauty is in the eyes of the beholder, in this case, there was almost perfect agreement among the researchers in their rating the attractiveness of each spouse. In other words, if one researcher rated a spouse as a 10, it was highly likely that the other researchers had the same rating. The researchers called this an objective attractiveness score.

It seems that being objectively attractive has a different impact on the relationship, depending on whether you are a man or a woman. Attractive wives behaved more positively and supportive during their interactions with their husbands. They listened more, nodded supportively, offered help to their partner, and encouraged them.

But attractive husbands behaved more negatively during the ten-minute discussions. They were more likely to blame their wives or criticize them, and in some cases, even ignore them. They were also less satisfied with their marriages.

Why did attractiveness affect behavior differently for men and women? Evolutionary psychologists say an attractive man feels that they have more short-term mating opportunities, which can make them feel less committed to their current relationship. As a result, they also feel less satisfied. Women, on the other hand, aren't as negatively affected by attractiveness because they view it as less important in a long-term relationship.

Attractiveness as a starting point for a relationship has mixed benefits. For men, an attractive mate signals a good mate. However, they may feel less of a need to commit to that relationship. For women, attractiveness in a mate does not appear to be a critical factor when looking for a suitable long-term relationship.

But interestingly, as the relationship develops, that initial attraction is less important. Instead, relative attractiveness makes a difference in how you interact with your spouse. If you view them as attractive (regardless of the "objective" attractiveness rating), you are more likely to behave in a positive and supportive way with them. This pattern is true for both men and women.

Finding Your Type

So if attraction isn't everything, how can women best evaluate a relationship fit?

"Ask Aunt Tracy. She can tell you whether Josh is a good guy." My brother glanced sideways at me and grinned as he leaned up against the kitchen counter, sipping his coffee. His fifteen-year-old daughter looked surprised. I'm pretty sure my brother was trying to deflect any potential pushback that was sure to come if he told his daughter that Josh is probably not the right guy for her.

Josh is an artist. A musician. He writes songs on the spur of the moment. He has a mop of sandy colored hair, which with one flick seems to elevate his status of coolness. Josh is also flaky and unreliable. He makes plans and then cancels at the last minute. But it is hard to be mad at him because, well, he has that hair.

Telling a teenage girl that there is more to a suitable suitor than good hair is tricky business. And not one that I was about to embark upon on a Saturday morning. So I grinned back at my brother and said to my niece, "Josh sounds nice."

My brother wasn't so easily deterred. "Ask her the questions," he said. "The five things."

Ah, the list of five things. So there is a list that makes a difference for the *longevity* in a relationship. And it is largely similar for men and women.

Which of these traits do you value in a partner?

- is reliable, can always be counted on
- assumes the best about people
- is fascinated by art, music, or literature
- is dominant, acts as a leader
- is funny but moody

Have you heard of the Big Five personality traits? Which traits did you select for a partner? I asked this same question to my followers on social media, and here is what it looked like, in the same order as the previous list:

- **Conscientiousness:** Is reliable, can always be counted on— selected by 60 percent of people (number one trait that both men and women valued in my social media survey)
- **Agreeableness:** Assumes the best about people—selected by 24 percent of people
- **Openness to experience:** Is fascinated by art, music, or literature—selected by 11 percent of people
- **Extroversion:** Is dominant, acts as a leader—selected by 5 percent of people
- **Neuroticism:** I didn't include this trait on my social media survey. People who are neurotic do have positive traits that can be attractive. They often have a quirky sense of humor and are self-deprecating, but they can also be self-conscious, become stressed easily, and be overly dependent in a relationship.

We each have a type: a *personality type*. The type we are attracted to is similar to our own personality. We may think that couples act like each other because they spend time together and grow old together. While that can play a role, a much better explanation comes from the choice that we make at the start of a relationship. It may be intentional, or it may be a "gut feeling," but we gravitate toward people whose personality resembles ours. This tendency is what sociologists call "assertive mating." There is one exception for when finding a mate with similar personality traits is less optimal and that is for extraversion. Women who are introverted and seek out men who are extroverted tend to experience more long-term benefits than those who are matched on levels of extraversion.[11]

Personality Traits across the Lifespan

How would you answer these questions?

- Do you confide in your partner?
- How often do you and your partner quarrel?

Those questions, along with thirty other questions, come from a survey called the Dyadic Adjustment Scale. It measures relationship satisfaction by exploring how often you agree (or disagree!), how connected you both are, and how affectionate you are with your partner.

Researchers from Simon Fraser University looked at 125 heterosexual couples in their fifties, sixties, and seventies. On average, these couples had been married around thirty-four years, and over 80 percent had been married only once. About two-thirds of the couples stated that they were happier in their relationship than the average couple.

Both partners answered personality questions from the Big Five personality test, like the ones you answered earlier. They rated their own personality traits, as well as their partners. It turns out that some of these traits are better than others if you want your relationship to last. Here is what the study found about ideal (and not so ideal!) relationships for both men and women.

1. *One personality trait that predicts relationship dissatisfaction is neuroticism.* This pattern has been consistently reported in both marital satisfaction and stability of the relationship. Highly neurotic partners tend to be moody, get upset easily, and can be self-conscious. They tend to be highly reactive to stress and are more likely to experience negative emotions (sadness, anger, and so on). They are also more likely to project these feelings onto a partner, which can create friction in a relationship.

   But neuroticism does have its positives. They are sensitive and aware of their partner's needs in ways that other people might not be. They can also be more aware of other people's feelings (usually because they want to be aware of the situation so they can prepare for any perceived threats). As a result, you may find yourself attracted to someone who has neurotic traits.

2. *Agreeableness is a powerful factor for marital satisfaction.* Agreeable people are optimistic and positive; they generally believe in the good in people and are more likely to trust people more. One of the key reasons this trait matters in a relationship is because agreeableness plays an important role in conflict resolution. People who are agreeable are more likely to seek out cooperative ways to

solve a problem, accept input from their partner, and be willing to work together as a team. Happy couples tend to be partners who are similar in their levels of agreeableness. But keep in mind that agreeable people may struggle to assert their needs. If you are with an agreeable person, be mindful of their needs too, especially because they may not always express them.

3. *Conscientiousness is most strongly linked to satisfaction in marriage.* A person scoring high in conscientiousness is usually highly self-disciplined and organized. They are also dependable and will stick to their commitments. This trait becomes more important the longer a couple has been together because a person scoring high in this trait is often willing to work hard at their relationship, especially during major changes, like empty nesting and retirement.

   For women, looking for conscientiousness in a mate can be a positive indicator for long-term satisfaction. If you are in your twenties and thirties, this may show up in your potential mate looking like workaholism, perfectionism, or even obsessive-compulsive tendencies. But this trait seems to mellow out as you age and is a good indicator that the person is willing to work to keep your relationship healthy.

It is important to remember that when it comes to personality traits and their impact on relationship satisfaction, the traits work symbiotically in a person. For example, someone who is high in neuroticism but high in conscientiousness can turn their anxiety into a positive and healthy outlet. Their sense of self-control motivates them. Likewise, high agreeableness can buffer against high neuroticism, which means the person may be less contentious or conflict-seeking in a relationship.

Summary: Women look for different things than men at the start of a relationship. They tend to seek out someone who is financially stable. But if you are a financially independent woman, it would be better for your long-term happiness to look for someone whose personality matches yours. For tips to move from the start of a relationship to a long-term bond, read the next chapter.

Think Like a Girl

1. **Look for important personality traits.**

   Look for a partner who is similar to you in his social needs, or mirrors your own level of introversion or extroversion.

2. **Conscientiousness and agreeableness are also traits to look for if you want to be more satisfied in your relationship long-term.**

Four

The Bonding Brain

Understanding the Power of Oxytocin

I have always wondered what it would be like to be able to turn off the craving for companionship, that need to connect or to bond with someone. I could say this curiosity comes from a purely psychological interest. But that wouldn't be true. Like Jim Carrey's character in the movie *Eternal Sunshine of the Spotless Mind*, we each have had a piece of what we call our "heart" broken. However, it is not really our heart that is affected, but rather our brain. And it starts at birth.

It Begins with a Touch

The moment a mother meets her child, her brain releases a neurotransmitter that helps her form an intense bond with her child.

Myth:

Women crave bonding in relationships more than men.

Studies show that mothers with high levels of oxytocin in the first month postpartum are more likely to coo and sing songs to and cuddle with their babies. This touch helps them bond.

The reverse is true too. When mothers of premature infants aren't given the opportunity to touch or hold their babies, they can experience difficulty in bonding. But a simple action like a massage or kangaroo care (skin-to-skin) with their infant can promote a closeness.

Women are hardwired with oxytocin. It helps during labor (it is even injected to induce contractions during labor), breastfeeding (when a baby latches on to the mother's breast), and bonding, as you just read.

Oxytocin plays an important role in bonding even in your romantic relationships. How would you answer these questions?

- Do you feel safe when the other person is nearby and responsive to your needs?
- Do you feel insecure when the other person is not accessible?
- Do you both share discoveries with each other?

Those questions could relate to your relationship with your mother. They could also relate to your relationship with your significant other. That is exactly what researchers from a British university noticed: the relationship between infants and caregivers and the relationship between adult romantic partners share many common features, just like in the questions you answered.[1] As a result, they suggested that our romantic relationships as adults are similar to the relationships with our parents—they are attachments, and we learn the ropes from an early age. We learn how to trust and how to interact. And those relationships leave us feeling safe and protected or unsafe and unprotected. This bond does not just have a fleeting impact. Take a look at the following statements.

Think about your past and present relationships with people who have been especially important to you, such as family members, romantic partners, and close friends.[2] Choose a statement that reflects how you generally feel in these relationships.

1. I find it relatively easy to get close to others and am comfortable depending on them and having them depend on me. I don't often worry about being abandoned or about someone getting too close to me.
2. I am somewhat uncomfortable being close to others; I find it difficult to trust them completely, difficult to allow myself to depend on them. I am nervous when anyone gets too close, and often, partners want me to be more intimate than I feel comfortable being.
3. I find that others are reluctant to get as close as I would like. I often worry that my partner doesn't really love me or won't want to stay with me. I want to merge completely with another person, and this desire sometimes scares people away.

Statement one refers to a *secure* attachment style: As an adult, you are comfortable depending on others and find it easy to get close to others. As a child, your parent/caregiver was likely responsive to your emotional needs and had positive interactions with you. As a result, you had a secure base from which you could explore and understand your surroundings. This allows you to trust people, you typically don't feel abandoned, and you feel a healthy sense of self-worth.

In a relationship, a person with a secure attachment style feels comfortable expressing their emotions. In conflict, they are able to focus on the issue, rather than attack the person. They also feel secure on their own, as well as with a partner.

Statement two refers to an *avoidant* attachment style: As an adult, you are reluctant to get close to other people, yet tend to be overly dependent on others. As a child, your parent/caregiver was likely aloof or distant and would rebuff your attempts to get close. As a result, you learned to suppress the need for intimacy to avoid rejection.

What does this look like in a romantic relationship? A person with an avoidant attachment style will be less likely to let themselves open up or be vulnerable in a relationship. They express a strong need for independence, to the point of pushing away a potential mate, maybe expressing statements like, "I need my space." They may also exclude their partner from their other activities, even in social situations.

Statement three refers to an *anxious/ambivalent* attachment style: As an adult, you are uncomfortable with closeness with others and have a difficult time trusting people. As a child, your parent/caregiver was likely inconsistent or overbearing in showing you love and affection. As a result, you likely felt anxious because you found it difficult to predict how your caregiver would respond to your emotional needs.

In this attachment style, the person is often unsure or insecure in their relationship. This results in them clinging on more strongly or becoming demanding or possessive of their partner's time. They are more likely to interpret their partner's behaviors in light of their own insecurities. For example, if their partner spends time with their friends, the person with an anxious attachment style will likely think, "They don't really love me, because they don't want to spend time with me."

Bonding in a relationship is, in a way, an attachment. You form an attachment with another person. If you don't know why you behave the way you do, you may end up repeating patterns of attachment that aren't healthy.

The attachments we form with our parents during childhood set the stage for the types of romantic attachments we create as adults. As adults, the qualities we seek in long-term relationships often match the caregiver qualities we saw in our parent (usually your mother): the warmth, the attentiveness, the sensitivity to our needs. When we see those in a potential partner, we consider those traits desirable.

Truth:

Early childhood attachments can make a big impact on adult romantic relationships, for both men and women.

The good news is that these attachment styles are not fixed. Psychologists suggest that the infant-caregiver attachment style teaches you a script of how to bond with someone but that you can change your behavior. So if you find yourself displaying attachment behaviors that aren't optimal, you can seek help to adjust those behavioral patterns.

Attachment styles impact romantic relationships differently for women and men.

For women, the *avoidant* attachment has a much bigger

impact on relationship satisfaction than an anxious attachment. In other words, the less avoidant they are, the more satisfied they feel in their romantic relationship. Why does avoidant attachment make such a difference for women? The researchers suggest that women find it more important to be able to share their feelings with their partner when they are in a relationship.[3] But if you have an avoidant attachment style, then you will find it difficult to foster a closeness with your romantic partner. As a result, it is difficult for you to trust or bond with your partner, leading to a dissatisfaction in your relationship.

But for men, *anxious* attachment and *avoidant* attachment have a similar impact on their relationship satisfaction. What does that mean for men? The researchers suggest that the anxious attachment is a clue that men find it more important than women to feel cared for by their partner. For example, men find it more important in a relationship to feel that their partner won't abandon them.

This feeling about abandonment is twice as important for men as it is for women. And its roots start as young as early childhood. One study that followed children from six years old up to twenty-one years old found that a feeling of abandonment persisted over the years.[4] In other words, if a child feels a sense of abandonment when they are six years old, they carry that through into adulthood, even into their romantic relationships.

From a Touch to a Hug

Whether you grew up with a secure, avoidant, or anxious/ambivalent attachment style, your ability to bond and create a lasting bond depends on something more biological—that hormone known as oxytocin. You have the ability to increase it.

It was all very theatrical. Paul Zak walked onto the stage, his right hand raised for effect. Then he sprayed something into the air. It was an elixir of sorts. Not quite the fountain of youth, but perhaps something better. Something that offered the promise of an end to all the ills that were unleashed when Pandora's box was opened. The promise of a new era—where people are more trusting, generous, and loyal. That is a tall order for a hormone. Oxytocin is often affectionately referred to as the "cuddle hormone." Economist and researcher Paul Zak suggests that hugs can release oxytocin. As a nonhugger myself, I was skeptical about Zak's theory, especially since he is an economist. But his work on hugging is in good company. Family therapist Virginia Satir said, "We need four hugs a day to survive, eight hugs to keep us as we are, and twelve hugs to grow."

While Satir had the right idea, research suggests that the length of the hug matters more than the number of hugs. Almost two hundred people were given the stressful task of public speaking, while being evaluated. But before this, half the group had the benefit of a twenty-second hug from their partner, while the other half just rested quietly on their own. Both men and women showed lower stress levels; having a supportive partner hug them for twenty seconds decreased stress.[5]

It seems that women especially benefit from a hug because female hormones enhance its effects. In a somewhat unusual study, Japanese researchers used a cushion to explore the impact of a hug.[6] They placed female participants into two groups. In one group, the participants talked to a stranger on the phone for fifteen minutes. Now, here is where it got interesting. The second group also talked to a stranger. But they had their conversation while hugging a human-shaped cushion that doubled as a phone. They called the cushion a Hugvie.

Even a cushion in the form of a hugger was enough to lower stress levels. Hugging while talking is much better for your stress levels than just talking alone. Stress levels were measured by checking cortisol levels from both blood and saliva samples. It may seem odd that a cushion is able to have such an impact. The Japanese researchers think it has to do with the hug posture itself. The way you open up your arms to create space could be instrumental in reducing your cortisol levels.[7] Maybe Zak was right after all. A hug is a powerful thing.

I recently experienced the power of a hug. For as long as I can remember, I have been engaged in public speaking. My first foray into this was in second grade. I participated in a statewide storytelling competition. I practiced every day in front of the mirror, my mother coaching me to put the intonations and emphases in the right places. On the big day of the competition, I remember standing on stage in my costume that my grandmother made for me, looking at everyone's faces. My mother, anticipating that I would be nervous and possibly freeze up, told me to imagine those faces as cabbages. It worked! As I opened my mouth to start my story, the image of rows and rows of cabbages sitting there seemed to dispel my nervousness.

Over the years, the content of my speaking has changed. Now instead of stories, I get to share my research with others. But my mom's tip stuck with me. Especially on one summer afternoon. I was keynote speaker at a conference for women from Fortune 500 companies. It was my first time doing such an event, and the speaker before me was the cofounder of HGTV. The pressure was on! The audience would definitely be expecting a dynamic and entertaining presentation. Suddenly the cabbages-instead-of-faces trick wasn't working.

My presentation was in Jacksonville, where I live. All through lunch, I kept looking at my watch and counting down to my presentation in my head. Then I felt a hand on my shoulder. I looked up. A friend had stopped by. "I know today is a big day. I can't stay, but I came to give you this." And she gave me a big hug. I don't know how she knew. But in that moment, I felt all my nervousness slip away. I had a great time on stage.

That hug from my friend did indeed decrease my stress level before my public speaking.

Hugs and Oxytocin in Romantic Relationships

Imagine that you and your loved one are having a conversation. You are talking about a recent vacation you went on. Every so often you laugh at a shared memory and squeeze your loved one's hand. They look back at you, and for a moment you both say nothing because you instinctively know what the other is thinking.

But this is no usual conversation between lovers. Not with the video camera in the corner or the audio recording equipment on the table. Researcher Ruth Feldman and her colleagues invited sixty couples who were within the first three months of their relationship to their comfortable lab. With the help of the recording equipment, they were able to observe how the couples interacted with each other as they talked about a fun experience.

The more they shared positive interactions, like affectionate touches, expressing positive emotions, and sharing concerns together, the higher their oxytocin levels.[8]

The cynic may say that these elevated oxytocin levels are just the result of "new love," a heady combination of novelty and excitement. But when the researchers brought some of these romantic pairs back into the lab six months later, their oxytocin levels remained high. The researchers stated that their oxytocin levels were similar to those expressed in a parent-child bond. Even Feldman was surprised. She said, "The increase in oxytocin during the period of falling in love was the highest that we ever found."[9] It was also double the levels she had previously recorded in pregnant women, which is a peak time for oxytocin, as it prepares a mother to bond with her newborn.[10]

Oxytocin levels at the start of a relationship are a good indicator of the staying power of a relationship. It was a telling sign of which couples would last until six months later. They touched each other more, they laughed together, and they finished each other's sentences. Interestingly, no difference existed between men and women's oxytocin levels. They both operated symbiotically: one partner's oxytocin levels predicted the level of positive engagement and touch in the other.

Feldman and her colleagues called this a "feedback loop": the more affection was expressed, the more it was reciprocated, and the more invested the couple felt in the relationship. She says, "Oxytocin can elicit loving behaviors, but giving and receiving these behaviors also promotes the release of oxytocin and leads to more of these behaviors."[11] It works in a beautiful, positive circular fashion: when you give love, you receive love, which makes you want to keep giving love. And it works the same for men and women.

Hug it out. Hugging while talking is much better for your stress levels than talking alone. Take twenty seconds and hug your partner to create that feedback loop and boost your oxytocin. The more you express physical affection, the more positive you will feel about your partner. . . . It can even help you through conflict.

Truth:

Regardless of your attachment style, you can increase bonding with your partner with a hug.

Oxytocin in Conflict

What was the last thing you and your significant other argued about? I am writing this chapter during the COVID-19 pandemic in 2020, and as a frequent contributor to the affiliate TV networks, I was asked to talk about how relationships are being taxed as a result of the stay-at-home and work-from-home mandates. Couples who are used to having their space and independence are now finding themselves in close and constant quarters.

One couple talked about how they were arguing about how much tuna to put in a tuna melt sandwich. "We had our first big blowup yesterday. I was in a really bad mood 'cause quarantine hit me and all I wanted to do was have time alone to cook. And Miranda was like, 'I want to help you,' and it really pissed me off. We were making tuna melts, and she added more tuna to my sandwich. . . . I was like, 'Why are you trying to [bleep] with this sandwich?' . . . As it was happening, I thought, 'This is so stupid. I'm not mad about this sandwich at all.' We hugged to resolve it."[12]

Conflict in relationships is probably the last thing you associate with attachment and closeness. But Beate Ditzen from the University of Zurich, Switzerland, disagrees.[13] She brought forty-seven heterosexual couples into the lab for a double-blind study (which means that neither the couples nor the researchers know who is receiving a particular treatment). One partner sprayed five puffs of oxytocin up their noses, while the other sprayed a placebo instead. If you think that a nose spritz sounds somewhat invasive, it is. But it also ensures that the oxytocin reaches the brain.

Forty-five minutes later, the couples were asked to talk about a disagreement or fight, like how they spent their free time or who did the housework. The timer was set for ten minutes, and the couples were left alone in a room and videotaped.

After the conflict discussion, participants were asked to evaluate their disagreement on several levels: how stressful was the fight, how positive were they and/or their partner during the fight, how negative were they and/or their partner during the fight, and did they and/or their partner come up with a solution. Then Ditzen asked them to spit. She wanted to measure their salivary alpha-amylase, an enzyme directly related to stress in social situations. That little spray of oxytocin made a difference.

But it wasn't the same for men and women.

When women received that spritz of oxytocin, they showed lower stress and wanted to *tend and befriend*. This resulted in their quieting down and displaying less "demand behaviors," which may unintentionally push their partner away. In a conflict, you may find that you talk louder and demand more, especially if you feel that your voice isn't being heard. Unfortunately, this behavior is counterproductive and often results in a man withdrawing from the conflict. But a little oxytocin can shift your response to a quieter one, and this shift can resolve the conflict.

With the men who received the spritz, they showed a spike in their stress levels. Yet, somewhat counterintuitively, they turned into better communicators when discussing the fight with their partner. They smiled more, showed more eye contact, and even talked more openly about their feelings (the holy grail of conflict resolution in relationships)!

Why did oxytocin have this remarkable and unexpected effect on the men? According to Ditzen, men tend to withdraw from their partner when they are in conflict. This results in a breakdown in communication and ultimately dissatisfaction with the relationship for both sides. But oxytocin results in higher emotional arousal, as evidenced by higher levels of the social stress marker in their saliva. As a result, they were more engaged and communicative with their partner, even when discussing a tricky topic, like a recent fight.

So if you don't have oxytocin spray on hand (kidding), a twenty-second hug can also elevate your oxytocin levels. Instead of trying to "talk it out," a more effective strategy may be to *stop* talking and hug instead.

Oxytocin in Love

When you are lost in the eyes of your loved one, wondering if the feeling of euphoria will last forever, you are not alone. Psychologists have wondered the same thing as well. One view is that the heady romantic love of a new relationship slowly develops into a companionship, where you enjoy each other's company and share interests but don't have that same burning passion for each other. Some psychologists have gone as far as to speculate that passion in a long-term relationship is a red flag because one party is over-idealizing their partner. Passion in long-term relationships has even been thought to reflect pathological tendencies (thank you, Freud!).

Psychologists Helen Fisher and Arthur Aron decided to put these views to the test. They recruited close to twenty people, average age fifty-three (ranging from thirty-nine to sixty-seven), who had been married on average for twenty-one years to someone of the opposite sex and were sexually active about twice a week. About half the people were in a first marriage for both partners, while the others were in marriages where one or both partners had been previously divorced.[14]

Participants were shown photos of their partner, a familiar acquaintance, and a close, long-term friend as a comparison. The friend was someone with whom the participant had a close, positive, interactive (but not romantic) relationship, and the participant knew them for about as long as their partner. Fisher reported two new, ground-breaking findings.

1. Long-term romantic love is similar to early-stage romantic love, at least in the brain. Partners showed similar levels of dopamine in the same brain areas (ventral tegmental area) that drive reward and motivation to pursue a goal. Interestingly, this pattern of activation was linked to their reported passionate love scores: the more in love they reported feeling, the greater the activation of dopamine in these areas. This means that the more in love they felt, the more rewarded they were in the brain. In

contrast, they didn't show these same patterns of activation when they were shown a photo of a close friend or familiar acquaintance.

2. The partners showed brain activation similar to maternal attachment when they looked at their partner's photo. This means we want to form bonds with a partner. We seek out closeness with someone in a meaningful way, and in a way that replicates our first close contact bond that provided support and nourishment. Interestingly, researchers suggest that it takes about two years for us to form an attachment bond, which is why newlyweds don't show this same level of brain activation.[15]

This long-term romantic love is so powerful that it is like a painkiller! The same research team, Helen Fisher and Arthur Aron, discovered that couples who have been married on average for twenty-one years showed brain activation in opioid brain regions, which manage anxiety and pain and even depression. Interestingly, this benefit has not been found in couples who are newly in love.

Truth: **Long-term love creates deep bonds for both women and men.**

Being in a long-term committed relationship has the capacity to make a partner feel a greater sense of calm and even relieve pain!

What's one secret to having a long-term romantic bond? It's called the *positive illusory bias.* This refers to our tendency to perceive our own relationship as having more positive qualities and fewer negative traits, compared with our friends' relationships. It can even refer to the tendency to view your partner in a more favorable light than they view themselves. You think more highly of your partner's virtues and minimize their faults. If you see stubbornness in your partner, you may perceive it as integrity rather than egocentrism.

In the beginning of your relationship, this can have a tremendous positive effect. You are more likely to feel satisfied in your relationship for longer, and your relationship will likely last longer. It is also an important approach to stave off the inevitable threats to a relationship, like conflicts of interests, different approaches to solving problems, and so on. For example, when your partner behaves in a way you don't like, the positive illusory bias makes you less likely to seek revenge and more likely to be accommodating to them. When there is a conflict of interest in decision-making, you are also more likely to sacrifice your own interest for your partner's interest.

A positive illusory bias has value beyond conflict resolution and relationship satisfaction. Researchers suggest that your partner could also use your positive view of them as a template for change. And it appears that there is a difference of how men and women practice this: women (both dating and married) tend to have a more positive view of men than vice versa.[16] Overall, the positive illusory bias results in the health and long-term stability of your relationship because you view your partner positively and, as a result, are more likely to invest in it and work toward its success.

Oxytocin in Men

Oxytocin also plays a role in keeping men loyal in a relationship. If you are worried that your romantic partner may stray from the relationship, maybe a hug is the answer.

In Ditzen's experiment, they recorded the couples' conflicts using the "magic ratio." According to relationship researcher John Gottman, the magic ratio is a 5:1 ratio of positive interactions to negative interactions. For every negative comment or feeling, there should be five positive ones between you and your partner. Couples in stable and fulfilling relationships do this. They share more positive words and actions with each other than negative ones.

Researchers from Germany put a group of young heterosexual men to the test. Half of them received three puffs of oxytocin delivered via a nasal spray, while the other half received three puffs of a saline solution, as a control spray. They were introduced to a beautiful female researcher whose job it was to smile and ask them questions. But let's be honest, who pays attention to the questions when they're distracted by an attractive person?

Some of the men were single, while others were in a monogamous relationship. As it turns out, if the man had oxytocin sprayed up his nose, he was more likely to keep his distance from this attractive woman. About four to six inches more likely. And it happened only with the men who were in a relationship.[17]

Why? Proximity is a signaling behavior: it lets the other person know you're interested. And true enough, the men kept the extra distance only from the female researcher, not from the male researcher. The spritz of oxytocin reminded men of their bond with their partner. It very likely activated feelings of trust and attachment. As a result, they avoided signaling any interest to the woman by keeping a physical distance from her. The researchers found the same pattern in the men's behavior even when they showed them photographs of attractive women!

Summary: Women are hardwired with oxytocin. It peaks during key bonding activities, like labor and nursing. Oxytocin is often affectionately referred to as the "cuddle hormone." Women and men can use physical touch, such as a twenty-second hug, to boost their oxytocin levels, helping to resolve conflict and create a long-lasting bond.

Think Like a Girl

1. **Avoid avoidance in your romantic relationships.**

   If your parent or caregiver was emotionally unavailable or unresponsive to your needs as a child, then you are likely to have an avoidant attachment style. But you can rewire your attachment style. Recognize that you are more likely to interpret stress as personal, even if your partner is sharing a stressful event that happened to them. Also, those with an avoidant attachment style tend to overthink. Choose date activities that are novel so that you are more likely to be present and in the moment.

2. **Develop independence if you have an anxious attachment style.**

   If you have an anxious attachment style, you may play games or manipulate your partner (like ignore their calls or do things to make them jealous) to get their attention or the emotional assurance you need. First, recognize that the anxious attachment type often seeks out the avoidant attachment person because the relationship cycle validates their fear of abandonment. Be aware of when you are codependent in a relationship and may be using other people to regulate your emotions instead of self-regulating. Seek therapy to help you work through this effectively.

3. Hug it out.

Hugging while talking is much better for your stress levels than just talking alone. Take twenty seconds and hug your partner! It creates a feedback loop: the more affection is expressed, the more it is reciprocated, and the more invested a couple feels in the relationship. Long-term romantic love can be similar to early-stage romantic love: the more in love you feel, the more rewarded you are in the brain (with dopamine!). Long-term romantic love also mimics a maternal bond as you form a closeness with someone and can be so powerful that it is like a painkiller.

4. Use the magic ratio.

The magic ratio is a 5:1 ratio of positive interactions to negative interactions. For every negative comment or feeling, there should be five positive ones between you and your partner. Make it an intention to measure out your interactions with your partner. Maybe you need to keep a tally to start. At the end of the day, look to see if you have the magic ratio in place in your interactions.

5. See your partner with rose-colored glasses.

Positive illusions can help you go the distance. The positive illusory bias makes you more likely to view your partner in a favorable light. As a result, you become more willing to accommodate them and sacrifice your own interests when dealing with conflict. This results in a stable, long-term relationship. To cultivate a positive illusory bias, think of their trait in a positive light. If you find your partner is stubborn, try thinking of it as integrity rather than egocentrism.

Part Three

The Intelligent Brain

Five

Liar, Liar, Brain on Fire

Why Women Lie and Why It Matters

Abigail stared directly at the small white card on the table in front of her. She blinked quickly, then glanced up briefly toward the door. For a moment, she reached her hand toward the card and then quickly drew it back. She shifted uncomfortably in her seat. She furtively looked toward the door again. This time she craned her neck to try to see as far around the corner as she could. She was pretty sure the coast was clear, but she couldn't be certain. She wrung her hands and then sat on them for a while. That white card was so close to her. All she had to do was flip it over. Just for a second. Enough for a quick glance.

Abigail was one of almost 140 school-aged children in a research study I ran. In a somewhat deceptive study, we played a game with six- and seven-year-olds where we set them up to be tempted to lie. Tellingly, the game is called the temptation paradigm. We presented the children with a set of questions written on cards. We told the children that they would receive a special prize for every correct answer. The questions were easy, such as, "What noise does a dog make?" (A: meow; B: quack; C: woof; D: moo). The right answer was written on the back of the card in colored ink (C: woof). There was also a random picture, like a boat or car, on the back of a card (more on this later). After the children had answered the questions, the researcher showed the answer on the back of the card.

For the last question, the researcher asked the children about a nonexistent cartoon character: "What is the name of the main character in the cartoon *Spaceboy*?" We made up the show *Spaceboy*. It doesn't exist. Here is where the temptation came in. Before the children could give their answer, the researcher stepped out of the room but first told the children not to turn over the card to look at the correct answer (which was Jim). The children were left alone. The card with the right answer was on the table in front of them. No one was looking. A hidden camera captured all the action.

When the researcher returned to the room, they asked the child what they thought the correct answer was. Since there is no cartoon called *Spaceboy*, the children could know that the correct answer was Jim only if they had looked at the back of the card. The answer *Jim* was written in green ink next to a picture of a monkey.

Abigail wiggled and squirmed and tried desperately to stop herself from turning over that card when the researcher left the room. Do you think she looked at the card? Of course she looked! And she lied about it when she was asked whether she had looked. In fact, 100 percent of the children lied and said they didn't look when the researcher left the room.

If Pinocchio Were a Real Child

Lying is a juggling act. We have to keep in mind what we want to say, what the other person knows, and what we think they think we know. Perspective taking is an important part of lie telling. To fabricate a convincing lie to someone, you have to imagine the person's mind, as well as create an explanation that fits with their mind. It also takes a unique kind of intelligence called *working memory* to process all the social cues that come at you fast when you are knee-deep in telling your lie. Think of working memory as "work"-ing to remember information.

Most children by the age of three or four are capable of simple denial. Consider the following exchange that every parent has experienced:

"Did you eat the cookies?"

"No."

"Are you sure?"

"Yes!"

"Why do you have crumbs on your shirt?"

"I don't know."

The child knows they are lying. The parent knows the child is lying. And the child probably knows that their parent knows they are lying too. But their working memory isn't able to think fast enough to come up with a plausible explanation for why they have crumbs on their shirt.

All this changes around six years of age. Working memory experiences a growth, and the child is able to develop a more sophisticated explanation for why cookie crumbs are on their shirt. They realize, "My mother will not believe I didn't eat the cookies if she can see crumbs on my shirt." When children tell sophisticated lies, they need to use their working memory to maintain their deception and avoid being caught. The bigger their working memory capacity, the more able they are to tell a convincing lie.

In my research, I found that children who are good liars are smarter than those who have trouble telling a convincing lie. In the study described previously with Abigail, I tested their working memory intelligence by showing the children a series of letters and asking them to remember which ones they had seen.[1]

The letter game seems straightforward. Until you have to remember three letters. And then four letters. And maybe even up to seven letters. The average six-year-old can remember and work with two pieces of information. In a lie situation, this translates to remembering what they did wrong and thinking of what to say. They don't have the working memory space also to think of the other person's (usually their parent's) perspective.

In my lab, I conducted a study of hundreds of individuals from five to eighty years old to find out more about how working memory grows at each age. The most dramatic growth is during childhood: working memory increases more in the first ten years than it does over the lifespan. Working memory capacity steadily increases up to our thirties. At that point, working memory reaches a peak and then plateaus. The average twenty-five-year-old can successfully remember about five or six items. As we get older, working memory capacity declines to around three to four items.[1]

The amount of information that working memory can process at each age has important implications when it comes to telling lies. I gave the children in my study two entrapment questions: "What color was the answer written in?" (green) and "What picture is on the back of the card?" (monkey). For many children, their working memory skills couldn't help them figure out that if they answered these questions correctly, the researcher would know that they had peeked at the back of the card.

That was Seth. His working memory was lower than the average six-year-old. His working memory was more like an average four-year-old. When the researcher asked Seth those entrapment questions, he immediately answered them correctly. He grinned broadly and asked if he could get his prize for getting them all right! His working memory was also not able to process that he just gave himself away: by answering those questions about the ink color and picture on the back of the card, the researcher now knew he had turned the card over when she left the room. His working memory also failed him when the researcher asked him how he knew the answer to the question about *Spaceboy*. Like the three-year-old who couldn't come up with a plausible explanation for why there were cookie crumbs on his shirt, Seth also spluttered as he tried to answer. He became flustered and tugged on his hair. He kept looking toward the door and finally said, "I don't know."

For some children, their working memory was extra strong. This allowed them to juggle the components of their lie, as well as keep the researcher's perspective in mind. They realized that if they claimed they didn't turn over the card when the researcher left the room, then they couldn't possibly know the answer to the entrapment questions. Instead, they gave wrong answers, like "red" and "lizard." I looked at how successful they were when they lied about this and compared it with their working memory score using the letter game described earlier in this chapter. As you can imagine, those who avoided entrapment had the highest working memory scores.

That's like Abigail. Her working memory was extra strong.

She had the working memory of a ten-year-old. This allowed her to take the perspective of the researcher when she was asked the entrapment questions. Her working memory helped her figure out that if she answered those questions correctly, then the researcher would know she had turned the card over and looked. Her strong working memory also meant she could easily manage more than two pieces of information when she was asked how she knew that the character of *Spaceboy* was Jim. She looked the researcher directly in the eye and calmly and confidently responded that she knew the answer because it was her favorite cartoon and she watched it every Saturday.

Abigail is honing her skills from an early age. After all, everybody lies. Extensive research exists on both the prevalence and the universality of lying behaviors. One study reported that one in five interactions includes a lie![2] But when it comes to who tells more lies, the common belief is that women lie less than men. Of course, this is a hotly debated topic. Neither side wants to take the prize on this one!

Myth:

Women are more honest and lie less than men.

If Pinocchio Had a Brain

To answer the question about who lies more, let's look under the hood. Lying has a bad reputation (and for good reason), but it is one of the biggest accomplishments of your brain. There are two key players in the brain:

1. Amygdala, the brain's emotional center: When you lie for personal gain, your amygdala produces a negative feeling that determines how far you will go in your lie-telling. Your amygdala is like your moral watchdog: it is filled with negative emotion when you engage in behaviors that you feel are wrong, like being dishonest. When people first tell a lie, the emotional response in the amygdala is high. In other words, it has a strong effect on them. Then if they tell a second lie and a third lie, the activity in the amygdala starts dropping. In other words, the more you tell lies, the more your brain adapts and becomes less emotionally sensitive to the deceptiveness. The more you lie, the more your watchdog quiets down and lets more lies through the gate.[3]

2. Prefrontal cortex, the executive part of the brain: The prefrontal cortex is the home of working memory, and it does the heavy lifting when you are lying. This is because a lie isn't based on actual memories, so your brain has to work hard to create a new story. Multiple brain imaging studies show that the prefrontal cortex is more active (measured by more blood flow to that area of the brain) when someone is lying.

The prefrontal cortex also shows differences in lying for men and women. In one study, people were put in a brain scanner and given 120 questions; 60 were personal questions (example: Do you have a sister?), and the other 60 questions were general information. They were asked to tell the truth about some of the questions and lie about others. As in the temptation paradigm game that I used with the children, the adults in this study had an incentive to lie—a prize at the end of the study. The best liars would receive forty euros (about US$45) for their sneakiness.[4]

As it turns out, women are better liars than men, at least according to their brain scans. When men were asked to lie about personal information, there was more activation in their prefrontal cortex. This means their brains worked harder when they were telling a lie. They also took longer to come up with a believable lie about personal information, compared with when they lied about general information.

In contrast, the women in the study did not show any differences in brain patterns when they lied. It also didn't take them any longer to tell a personal lie than a general lie. One explanation is that lying about personal information for women is less cognitively effortful because they do it on a regular basis. Social norms or expectations can mean women need to present themselves in a certain way and will engage in a few lies to do so. For example, women often lie about their age, their interests, or other personal information for fear of being judged or overlooked at work.

Truth:

Women are better liars than men.

If Pinocchio Were a Woman

What sorts of lies do women tell? Are they different from the lies men tell? Imagine this scenario:

> You own and operate a small number of luxury hotels in the region and want to complete an important real-estate negotiation. You want to build a high-rise hotel because the property is on a prime tourist spot. But the seller wants to sell the property to make residences. Here is the conundrum. Would you be honest and reveal your true intentions for the property (and risk losing the deal)? Or would you tell a little lie? After all, it's not up to the seller to decide how you choose to use the property.

Now imagine the same scenario, but this time you aren't acting for yourself but as an agent for someone else. Would that change how you negotiate with the seller? Your answer depends on whether you are a man or a woman, according to researchers from Northwestern University and Berkley University. They presented 160 participants, 50 percent of whom were female, with those scenarios. Here is what they found:

- Women are 45 percent more likely to lie when they are representing a client, compared with when they are representing themselves.
- Men typically behave similarly in both scenarios, though they are 15 percent less likely to lie for a client than for themselves.[5]

Women lie differently than men. They will lie *less* when they are lying about themselves. But they will lie *more* when they are asked to lie for someone else. This is called *prosocial lying*, and it is the bright side of lying. Prosocial lies are told for the benefit of someone else, to spare someone's feelings or even to help them feel a little better about themselves. These types of lies are often harmless or can even come from a "good place." After all, isn't it nice that you told Jenny that she looks great in her new dress and Michael that he did a good job singing karaoke? The outcome of both these prosocial lies is that the receiver feels good about themselves.

Truth:

Women lie for different reasons than men.

Contrast that with what psychologists call *antisocial lying*: lying to avoid punishment or lying for personal gain. This type of lying usually results in someone getting hurt. In one study in which people were asked to keep a diary of their interactions and lies for a week, everyday antisocial lies included these ones:

- Said I did not have change for a dollar.
- Told him I had done poorly on my calculus homework when I had aced it.
- Said I had been true to my girl.[6]

If Pinocchio Were a Girl

Men and women tell different types of lies. And it starts as early as preschool. I wanted to understand more about how prosocial and antisocial lying develops, so I recruited about thirty pre-school children and asked them to play a game. The goal was to shoot ten paper balls into a wicker basket on the ground. The paper balls were placed on the table in front of the child and could be used only once. Each paper ball was worth one point, and the child had to score a minimum of seven points to win a prize. We instructed the child to stand behind a clearly marked blue line approximately five feet behind the basket and not to cross the line or it would be considered cheating. A small concealed video camera captured the children's responses. Throughout all this, the researcher had their back turned away from the child and pretended to be busy with some papers. At the end of the game, the researcher asked: "Did you cross the blue line when you were playing?" Their self-reports were compared with the video footage and coded as lies or truths.

Next, the child watched an adult play the same game. They

had the same rules and opportunity to win a prize. We instructed the adult to intentionally step over the line and throw the balls multiple times in the child's presence. As before, the researcher remained in the room but pretended not to notice what was happening. At the end of the game, the researcher asked the child the same question: "Did the adult cross the blue line when they were playing?"

These preschoolers behaved similarly to the adults in the property negotiation study I described previously. The boys typically lied for themselves, while girls lied to protect the researcher. In other words, the boys were more likely to tell antisocial lies: they didn't want to be caught cheating! But the girls were less concerned about getting in trouble. They were thinking about the adult playing the game. They didn't want the adult to get in trouble. So they fudged the truth a little and said the researcher didn't cross the line even though they saw them do it.

Prosocial lying is more than "white lies" to please an adult. We now know that lying involves perspective taking and a certain kind of intelligence (working memory). Of all the types of lies you tell, prosocial lying is the zenith of lying if we rank lies from "bad" to "good." Why? Because it is highly motivated by empathy and compassion. When you tell a prosocial lie, it shows that you are prioritizing someone else's feelings (empathy) and are willing to risk a negative consequence to help them feel better (compassion). And it seems that, even from a young age, girls are developing this skill.

Girls grow up, and as adults, women continue this behavior of prosocial lying, even in everyday interactions, such as "That was a lovely dinner" or "You look great." It's not that women don't value the truth or think it isn't important. It's just that they value other people's feelings more.

So when you catch yourself about to tell a white lie or a whopper, know that, yes, your working memory is helping you out, but also pay attention to your amygdala. If you realize you've lied, even for prosocial reasons, consider what is happening in your brain. The more often you lie, the more you turn down the dial of your moral watchdog.

If Pinocchio's Nose Were Real

Can we trust people to tell the truth about lying? And if we can't, then do they have a "tell" that will reveal their true intent? Some will say that if someone looks away, you know they are lying. Others say fidgeting or playing with their hands is a giveaway. But a group of researchers from Spain thinks we don't need to know the tells that people display when they are lying. Because we have a far more telling tell. And it is one you can't control!

Here is how the researchers know. They gathered a group of participants and put them in two situations: 1) a high-stakes, mentally challenging scenario where half the participants lie and the other half are asked to tell the truth and 2) a low-stakes scenario where again half the participants are asked to lie, while the other half are asked to tell the truth.[7]

In both scenarios, participants sat in a thermography lab that captured infrared imaging of temperature changes. As it turns out, the childhood chant about liars and fire didn't quite get it right. When you tell a lie, something is on fire, but it isn't your pants. It's your nose! It is aptly called the "Pinocchio effect." The researchers reported that thermographic cameras resulted in an 85 percent accuracy rate in lie detection, and only one out of four false alarms.

Why the nose? This part of the face is most sensitive to changes in temperature. The researchers found that when people are highly anxious and have to think hard about their lie, their nasal temperature increases. But when they feel less anxious and don't have to think hard about their lie, their nasal temperature decreased. In other words, the more you have to think hard about your lie and the more anxious you are, the more likely your nose will be on fire.

Summary: Women are better liars than men, but for socially conditioned reasons. Brain activation patterns suggest that when women lie about personal information, it is not more effortful or harder than lying about general information. Maybe because we do it more! Women are also more likely to lie to protect someone. This pattern is found even in young girls, which means that from a young age, women learn how to navigate tricky situations in order to help someone else feel better.

Think Like a Girl

Before you are too hard on yourself for telling a white lie, recognize that lying is a sign of intelligence. Your working memory helps you process the social cues in front of you and keeps another person's perspective in mind. Here are some other things you can do to maximize this intelligence.

1. **Tell the truth with care.**

    Recognize that as a woman, you are more likely to engage in prosocial lying to protect another person's feelings. Part of that is taking a moment to adopt their perspective, which can be a good thing! But it is possible to step into another person's shoes, practice empathy, and tell the truth gently and with care. Twisting the truth, even for the "good" reason of avoiding hurting another's feelings, is not the only option.

2. **Listen to the lie watchdog.**

   The amygdala is your brain's emotional center, and there is often a strong emotional response when you do something you feel is wrong, like tell a lie. But the more lies you tell, the more your brain adapts, and the less emotionally sensitive your brain will be. So pay attention to your amygdala, trust it, and learn when to listen to it.

Six

The Creative Brain

Unleashing Your Unique Capacity for Creativity

Sarah Halstead shifts her weight from right to left as she stares into the camera. She is seated on top of a rustic wooden table in her backyard. Her tailored red blazer seems perfectly out of place. So does her well-coiffed blonde hair. "Oh, honey, you don't need a wide shot of this," she says as the camera pans down to reveal her pajama bottoms. She grins and keeps talking. "Just the waist up. It's one of the perks of this thing."[1] She's filming a bit to promote her segment for *All Together Now*, a livestreaming event to support the city of Los Angeles during the coronavirus pandemic.

Halstead joined Tim Allen, Jeff Bridges, and others for a show viewed in over seventy countries. Her self-effacing humor draws you in. Before long, that fifteen-second clip you started watching turns into an hour.

Halstead's new comedy show, *RVs and Cats*, is an

autobiography. A lady from Flint, Michigan, finds herself spinning her wheels in a job she doesn't like and married to a man who doesn't like her. So she buys a thirty-foot RV, packs her cat and suitcase, and sets off across the country without much of a plan. The show dropped at a perfect time. The world was pushed indoors due to shutdowns and social distancing requirements. Everyone was busy figuring out how many times they could rewatch a TV series before they were paralyzed by boredom.

Halstead's humor strikes a chord, and she works hard to connect with her audience. She tells me that if a joke doesn't work, it is better to own it: "Yeah, I didn't like that joke either," she'll confess onstage. That approach goes over well: "The audience loves when I acknowledge that a joke doesn't go over well. They like to be on the train with you. But there is a fine line. They don't like an amateur comic either; they like to feel that the comic is in control."[2]

Myth:

Women aren't as funny or creative as men.

If you were to pause for a minute to think of your favorite comedian or someone whom you find funny, chances are the person who comes to mind is a man. Comedy or any creative endeavor is tricky for a woman to navigate, largely because the prevailing view is that creativity is a male domain. And it is not in only male-dominated fields such as finance and architecture. It is even in how we perceive public speaking.

The Magic Ingredients of Creativity

In a unique study, researchers from Duke University used TED Talks as a measure of creativity. This study was of particular interest to me since I have given a TEDx Talk. The researchers asked people to watch one hundred TED Talks that had each garnered up to 30 million views. Topics included technology, entertainment, design, business, science, and global issues. Participants chose three words from the list below to describe each talk. Which of their words do you associate with creativity?

- ingenious
- confusing
- courageous
- fascinating
- funny
- informative
- inspiring
- long-winded
- persuasive
- unconvincing

The researchers calculated the number of times the participants used the word *ingenious* to describe a TED Talk. They used that word approximately 70 percent more for a talk given by a male speaker compared with a female speaker.[3] Halstead shares that she has heard all sorts of words used to describe her performance. Everything from genuine, relatable, and clever to badass. But never ingenious.

The same study showed that people think masculine traits like daring, decisive, and competitive are more important to the creative process. In contrast, stereotypically feminine characteristics like cooperative, nurturing, and supportive were much less associated with thinking outside the box. One explanation for why this view of male-female differences in creativity is so prevalent could be rooted in the way in which we are rewarded.

Rewards can motivate us. Usually, when you know you will receive a reward, you are more likely to repeat that behavior, like when you were paid to mow the lawn or babysit your younger siblings. But when it comes to creativity, it is not so simple. Offering a reward can undermine the creative process because you become fixated on getting the reward, which can make you lose interest in the task itself.

You shift from being *intrinsically motivated* (meaning you do because you want it or because you enjoy it) to being *extrinsically motivated* (meaning you do because you want the reward). Numerous studies show that when money or pizza parties are offered, people become disengaged from a creative task like art or music. In a task that involves creativity, it is better when you find inspiration from within, rather than from seeking a reward.

For Halstead, doing stand-up is itself rewarding. "It's euphoric when you get that kind of applause, when you feel the floor rumble. I'm always chasing that moment, and it's daunting and it's scary. It's like the adrenaline of skydiving and bungee jumping. Every time I put my little toe on that stage, I don't know how it's going to go. But it is such a nice feeling to have made people smile and laugh."[4]

Not all people view rewards equally. Girls are *less* creative when they know they will be evaluated, while boys are unaffected. The type of praise matters too, depending on whether you are a male or female. Here is how we typically praise children:

- **Girls:** We tend to praise girls for being "so smart" or "so clever" (ability praise). But it can have a big impact on their self-esteem. When you praise a child for their personal qualities, they connect it with their self-worth and view failure as a personal flaw and may think they are unworthy. When a child is praised for an ability, they may also struggle to deal with setbacks in the future. In fact, girls show more intrinsic motivation when they are given *effort* praise ("You did a great job").

- **Boys:** We tend to praise boys for their effort. Researchers from the University of Chicago and Stanford University found that this difference in how we praise can have long-term effects on a child.[5] They looked at both male and female toddlers and then followed up when they were eight years old. The toddlers who received praise for their efforts were not only better at solving difficult tasks, but they also believed they could change their outcome through hard work.

To boost your creativity, don't try to force creativity under an evaluation or performance setting. Instead, think of what you love about that particular project or activity. What motivates you to pursue that project? Make the creative process one that is fun and organic, rather than one that will be evaluated.

Truth:

Women are creative, just in different ways than men.

Turn On Your Network

Researchers from Indiana University explored the brain areas during creativity, investigating the strength of brain connections during a creative task.[6] The researchers found that the most creative people use parts of the brain that don't typically work together. Some parts of the brain are turned up, while others have to be turned down.

The frontal lobe is responsible for a lot of executive skills, like working memory (my area of research expertise), self-reflection, inhibition, and more. Some scientists have also attributed the frontal lobe as the seat of consciousness. But during the creative process, you need to turn down this part of the brain.

Is there a neurological difference in how men and women use their brain connections? Although neurological studies on this topic are sparse, some interesting differences exist in terms of efficiency and strength of the connections between the default mode network and the salience network.

- **Default mode network:** The brain's "idle state." This is when you are daydreaming and your mind wanders without any real purpose or intention. This part of the brain is in the frontal lobe and is involved in memory. It is important for brainstorming but can also leave you in a rut because you may revert to ideas that you have stored in your memory, resulting in something unoriginal.
- **Salience network:** This is the heavy hitter when it comes to creativity because its function is to sort through the ideas that the default mode network generates. After all, not every idea is worth pursuing, and your salience network helps you figure out which to keep and which to dump.

Men and women use their brains differently during the creative process.

Women tend to adopt a more generalized approach, drawing from different areas in the brain. This suggests a more diffuse way of thinking: when women are highly creative, they draw from different areas of the brain when they are coming up with an original idea.

Men tend to adopt a more localized approach, drawing from specific areas in the brain. When men are highly creative, there are more direct connections between the brain networks. This pattern suggests a more efficient system of processing information that makes use of "local knowledge" in the brain.

Ultimately what separates highly creative people (men and women) from those who are not is the way in which the parts of their brain work *together*. It is a synchrony between the brain networks that helps you think more creatively and flexibly—the back and forth between letting yourself daydream while still keeping an eye on sorting through the ideas that are germinating. Creative people are highly skilled at shifting between the daydreaming mode of thinking to the analytic mode.

To give your brain a chance to shift between modes, walk away from your ideas. Researchers from the University of Texas, Austin, found that even a quiet twenty-minute walk resulted in more creative ideas. Creativity is not instantaneous, and a short incubation period can unlock some original ideas. That is why some of the best "aha" moments come when you aren't thinking about the topic. When you step away from an idea you are stuck on, it gives your default mode network an opportunity to shine. This daydreaming state lets your brain flit from one thought to another, which can result in a creative idea.

For Halstead, she never plans to sit down and write a set. It happens almost unplanned, like when she is on her elliptical machine, listening to music, or as she puts it, "Rocking out to the White Stripes or Mary J. Blige."[7] She has even been sitting in traffic when an idea comes to her. Often she is immersed in the moment of an unrelated activity, like the time she was shopping for makeup. She found a blush collection with unusual names: Orgasm and Super Orgasm. Who chooses just Orgasm? Would she be an under-achiever if she chose that and not the Super version? Did they have a color called Almost There? Halstead pulled out her phone and wrote her comedy bit while standing in the makeup aisle.

A Brick and Creativity

You probably don't think a brick could help you be funnier or more creative, but play along with me. For two minutes, write down as many possible uses you can think of for a brick.

_____

_____

_____

_____

_____

_____

_____

_____

_____

I posed this same question to over 160 people from my research lab. Here is what they wrote:

- paperweight
- step stool
- break a window
- anchor
- oven
- mailbox

I posted the same question on social media. Here are their responses:

- paint on it
- write a wish and toss it in a lake
- burpees to shoulder press
- paint a smiley face and put in the yard for people to see as they walk by
- make music
- headstand on it

If you tried this activity, you probably agree that it is not as easy as it looks. Your default mode network was probably recruited to list things you are familiar with, like building-related activities. But your salience network may have swung you to the other side, where you came up with an original but implausible idea, such as using a brick as a camera to take a picture.

The brick question was first developed in 1967, and it may not seem creative to you. But it is very effective at weeding out the ordinary answers (build a house) from the original answers (headstand on it). Originality is one of the key criteria for creativity. The brick question tests creativity by asking you to take something familiar and come up with something novel.

A common definition of creativity is "divergent thinking." You may know it as "thinking outside the box." It is the idea that you can generate a potentially unlimited number of ideas or solutions. A bit of unpredictability exists in divergent thinking: sometimes you may end up with an idea that is implausible, but other times you might come up with a solution that is inspired and even groundbreaking. Many studies show that your ability to come up with an original use of a brick determines how creative you are in the real world, in both the arts and sciences. In other words, you are more likely to be innovative if you said a brick could be used to do a headstand on.

Divergent thinking is in contrast to *convergent thinking*, where you usually have one correct answer to a problem. When thinking in a convergent manner, you may start with multiple solutions but slowly and systematically narrow it down to the best one. If you like structure and rules, you are likely a convergent thinker.

In school, you learn that convergent thinking gets you the good grades. Think of a quiz or an exam during your school days. No matter how much you may have tried to argue with your professor, there is typically only one right answer. But in life, convergent thinking can often result in a set pattern of thinking. Using the same familiar solution to try to solve a new problem isn't what will set you apart in the workplace. But divergent thinking can help you break the mold.

Halstead agrees. As a stand-up comic, she tells me that "everyone has their own way." This sentiment reflects the premise of divergent thinking: There are many ways to tell a joke. The trick is knowing how to connect with your audience.

In comedy, surprise is key. Even TED speakers say so—at least the *ingenious* ones do! You don't get surprise in convergent thinking. You get surprise only in divergent thinking because the audience doesn't know which path you will take them down. Halstead uses this format in her comedy sets: premise → setup → punch line. She goes through a premise and then works through all the possible punch lines. The winner is always the one that has an element of surprise. "It's no fun if people can guess where the joke is going," she says. For her, that's the hardest part. When you dissect a joke, it's not always funny, but it should be surprising.

Why is surprise so fundamental in humor? Psychologists and even philosophers have explored this question. It is called the *incongruity principle*: the disconnection between our expectation and reality. When someone tells you a story, your brain has already jumped ahead to anticipate the ending. Your brain draws on similar previous experiences and has already created a road map of where the narrative is heading. As a result, you have an expectation of how the story will go. But the punch line violates that expectation. And that little surprise will hopefully draw a laugh.

Do women engage in divergent thinking more than men? That depends. In the brick test, there was no difference in original responses between men and women.[8] But an investigation of brain patterns during this task reveals that men and women use different strategies. Women typically use the language areas of the brain, related to speech processing and social perception. They draw on connections between the self and others. In contrast, men use brain regions related to declarative memory (knowledge about the world) and rule-learning and decision-making.

The Improv Brain or The Funny Brain

Let's play a game. It's called "yes and."

I will write a phrase. You finish it in a way that keeps the story moving forward.

> *Roses are red.*
> (Your turn) *Yes and . . .*

Anthony Veneziale, an improv expert with over twenty-five years of experience, played this same game as he lay on his back in a brain scanner. He had reached out to neuroscientist Charles Limb to collaborate on how the brain works during the creative process. Limb has done similar work with musicians, in part fueled by his own love of music.[9]

Veneziale started off with an initial scan to give the researchers a baseline of how his brain works. It took only five minutes. Then Limb used a functional MRI to take pictures of the active areas (increased blood flow) of Veneziale's brain when it was working hard during a particular task.

As Veneziale was lying in the fMRI scanner, he was given several common idioms and asked to improvise using "Yes, and" just like you did. He was riffing off the researcher's responses. Here is what they said:

> *Roses are red.*
> **Researcher:** Like the velvet curtains in the theatre.
> **Veneziale:** Yes, and the theatre is the magical
> dreamscape of your mind; Yes, and red velvet cake
> is my favorite.

Veneziale kept going. After this game, he played another improv game: "Take five seconds to come up with three things that fit into a given category." He responded rapid-fire back to the researcher.

Phone apps: "Tinder, Facebook, Volume"
Awards: "All of them? For me? Thank you."
Numbers: "1, 2, 3"
Colors: "Red, white, and blue"

Veneziale was one of several improv comedians that stepped into the scanner to help Limb understand the brain when it is being creative. While Limb is careful to note that you can't quite capture the magic of an improv moment inside a scanner, he did notice vast and measurable differences between the comedians who memorize their segments and the improv comedians.

When Limb had the comedians in the brain scanner, he found that the improv comedians showed strong activation in the areas of the brain that process language. In other words, they were quick to come up with a witty response thanks to all that extra blood flow to their brain's language center. That pattern was found only in the brains of the improv comedians. Because their comedy bit wasn't prerehearsed or committed to memory, they had to generate their humor spontaneously. And this activity uses language. Comedian Sarah Halstead says that her best comedic bits are the ones she wrote just before the show. "Those bits seem to get the biggest laugh compared to bits I have had in my arsenal for years."[10]

Limb found that it is not only comedy that activates the language center in your brain. Music does too. When he put Mike Pope, one of the world's best bassists in the brain scanner, he saw that his language center lit up as well! Music is a language. And even when you are a solo musician, it is a conversation with your audience. That communication is creative and expressive.

Limb is quick to add that we all engage in a highly creative process every day.[11] Talking! If you want to improve the creative networks in your brain, seek out conversations that are different from your usual daily topics. Even if you feel out of place at first, find people who have different opinions or skills in things you don't. The next time you stop for coffee, take some time to strike up a conversation with someone. Even if they are talking about the game last night that you have no interest in, make the effort to try to learn something new. Your creative brain will thank you.

If your creativity is lacking, your brain may need some new connections. Remember that your creative brain works best when it can draw from different things. Don't try to force a certain way of thinking. Imagine your brain like a web, and you drawing from different sections to come up with a creative idea.

Summary: Women are creative, just in different ways than men. Women draw from different areas of the brain when they are coming up with an original idea. Think of it as a *generalized* approach.

Think Like a Girl

Maximize your brain patterns and enhance your creative process with these tips:

1. **Skip the evaluation.**

   Keep your creative process fun and organic rather than one that will be evaluated. Think of the things you enjoy about your project rather than how your performance will be appraised.

2. Walk away from your ideas.

Creativity is not instantaneous, and a short incubation period can unlock some original ideas. Remember how we talked about the brain's default mode network, the brain's "idle state"? Step away from an idea that you are stuck on to give your default mode network an opportunity to shine.

3. Improve your divergent thinking skills.

One fun way to develop your divergent thinking is to brainstorm. Play games like the brick game. Challenge yourself to come up with novel and original uses of ordinary objects, like a brick or a pencil. You can even play this game with friends: the winner is the person with the most original uses for that object.

4. Have new conversations.

Seek out conversations that are different from your usual daily topics to improve your creative networks in the brain.

Part Four

The Feeling Brain

Seven

The Happy Brain

Habits for a Healthy and Happy Brain

I did not light a candle. But the hypnotic flame in the small glass on the altar was inviting me to do so. I gazed at it for a while. Then I bowed my head. I didn't have any words to say. Although I grew up saying the Lord's Prayer at bedtime, no supplication came to mind. So I just stood for a moment in silence. It seemed odd that I would find a moment of serenity surrounded by a throng of people, some talking in loud whispers, others taking covert selfies. Yet in that open room in St. Peter's Basilica, I felt a flicker of happiness.

I was in Rome for the summer as a visiting professor at one of the oldest universities in the world. I had been to Rome several times, but this time was different. In fact, it was one of the hardest summers. My marriage had recently ended, and I thought that accepting this position would be a good diversion from my personal turmoil, an opportunity to throw myself into my professional interests and the work that I'm passionate about. But many of the places reminded me of the times we had been there before as a couple.

"What makes you happy?" my colleague had asked me earlier that day. The question wasn't directed toward my personal pursuit of happiness. We were working on a research grant that investigated the factors that matter when it comes to mental health. Yet as we sat in his research lab reviewing scientific studies on the topic, I couldn't help but reflect on my own happiness.

I thought of author Gretchen Rubin's question as she spent a year chasing happiness: "Was it supremely self-centered to spend so much effort on my own happiness?"[1] We all want to be happy. It's even written in the US Constitution as an unalienable right: the pursuit of happiness. The focus on, maybe even obsession with, happiness seems to be uniquely Western. I spent my childhood in Malaysia. I don't ever recall a time when someone asked me whether I was happy. People asked if I studied hard, if I listened to my parents, if I was a good sister. Never if I was happy. Yet as an adult living in the US, I hear this topic come up often (and not just when I initiate conversation about it for research!).

What makes you happy?

Happiness for me may not be the same as it is for you. Recently, someone told me that happiness meant that they could retire in a few years and spend their days making furniture. Maybe one way to think of happiness is in the context of meaning. We experience happiness when we have the opportunity to pursue what is meaningful to us. Meaning is an existential question.

What do you find meaningful? I encourage you to reflect on this question as you read this chapter. Perhaps you will discover that what you spend your time on is not meaningful to you, and thus, you aren't experiencing happiness. Or perhaps you will find that what you spend your time pursuing is fulfilling and a source of happiness.

Think of the flip side of happiness as depression. Of course, various biological and social factors contribute to depression. But a big contributor stems from a *loss of control.* If you believe you are in control of the events in your life, even when faced with challenges, you will likely become proactive and take action to endure these difficult times.

Myth:

Women are unhappier (read: more susceptible to depression) than men.

On the other hand, some individuals believe they have little control over the events they experience, or that those events happen because of chance. These individuals will likely experience distress and become more passive in their behavior because they think their actions will not make a difference or change what is happening in their life. They eventually develop a sense of learned helplessness, a sense of powerlessness, because they believe their actions won't lead to a different outcome.

Which of these statements best describes how you feel?

a. Many of the unhappy things in people's lives are partly due to bad luck.
b. People's misfortunes result from the mistakes they make.

a. No matter how hard you try, some people just don't like you.

b. People who can't get others to like them don't understand how to get along with others.

a. I have often found that what is going to happen will happen.
b. Trusting to fate has never turned out as well for me as making a decision to take a definite course of action.

Locus of control is the idea that you have control over the events and experiences in your life. The theory of locus of control helps to explain, in part, why some people are able to successfully adapt to the demands of life, while others become vulnerable to depression.

If you chose more A statements, you have a strong *external* locus of control. This means you believe that what happens to you is the result of fate, or something that is not in your control.

If you chose more B statements, then you have a strong *internal* locus of control. You believe that the events in your life (good and bad) happen because of the decisions you made and the actions you took.

Having an internal locus of control does not mean you believe you can control events around you. Instead, it means you shift your focus to what you can control. This is a common coping strategy during stressful times: identify what events or actions are within your control and focus your energy on those. This simple strategy offers you meaning (and thus, some measure of happiness), even during difficult times.

Now, the myth is partially true. Women *are* twice as likely as men to experience depression. But depression is not a "normal" or expected part of being a woman. In other words, being a woman doesn't mean you will automatically experience depression.

A part of the brain called the locus coeruleus is responsible in part for producing a hormone called norepinephrine. A deficit of this hormone is related to depression, anxiety, and even trouble sleeping. And the female brain has three times more receptors associated with stress and depression, which can explain why we are more likely to be affected.

Truth:

Women are more susceptible to the blues than men but can learn ways to be happy.

If you are a woman affected by depression, one effective way to tackle your brain's neurochemistry is exercise. For example, one study found that exercise was as effective as medication.[2] Why does exercise work? It boosts norepinephrine, the brain neurotransmitter that is linked to depression. But if you are sad or depressed, it is often hard to be motivated. So break it into small steps. Start with one simple action. "I'll wear running shoes today." Research shows that wearing running shoes makes you more likely to exercise, compared to when you wear nonexercise shoes. As a clinical psychologist, I realize depression can be debilitating. It is important to seek treatment from your doctor or a therapist if you are experiencing depressive symptoms. You don't have to walk through this alone.

Happiness and You, the Agent

The gender gap in happiness may exist because of a difference in agency. Do you have agency at work? Do you have agency at home? For me, during the summer in Rome, I felt that I had agency at work. I love what I do. Any long hours or working weekends never felt onerous because I enjoyed work so much.

Home was a different story. I felt far less agency. Despite being intentional in starting my day with positive activities, like going for a run and writing down something I was grateful for, it still felt like a tremendous struggle. On some days even simple activities, like getting groceries, felt overwhelming. I felt like I couldn't get out of the car and into the store. I would tell myself that all I had to do was put my right foot out first and then my left one. I would repeat this till I found myself inside the grocery store.

How does this sense of agency (or lack of) affect your state of happiness? Read these statements.

Indicate how true each statement is of your experiences on the whole (1 = Not true at all; 5 = Completely true).

- My decisions represent my most important values and feelings.
- I strongly identify with the things I do.
- My actions are congruent with who I really am.
- My whole self stands behind the important decisions I make.
- The things I want or care about steadily inform my decisions.

Those five statements measure a sense of agency where the person feels like they are author of their own behavior. Men and women respond differently when it comes to mental health and happiness. For men, how they felt about those five statements made the biggest impact on their mental health. This means that when a man felt they were able to control and manage their actions and events in their life, or the more authorship they felt, the fewer depressive symptoms they experienced. In other words, when men have a sense of agency for their actions, they feel happier.

Here is where it gets interesting. Women in my study reported a similar sense of agency and control in their lives as the men in my study. Yet this didn't make a difference in their feelings of happiness. As a woman, it is not enough to feel that you are in control of your decisions. Something else makes a bigger impact on your state of happiness. Look at the following statements.

For each of the following statements, rate your level of agreement (1 = Strongly disagree; 5 = Strongly agree).

- My attention is often focused on aspects of myself I wish I'd stop thinking about.
- I always seem to be rehashing in my mind recent things I've said or done.
- Sometimes it is hard to shut off thoughts about myself.
- Long after an argument or disagreement is over with, my thoughts keep going back to what happened.
- I tend to "ruminate" or dwell over things that happen to me for a long time afterward.

Rumination is the word psychologists use to describe overthinking. Rumination matters when it comes to depression. Women are more likely to ruminate or keep replaying a distressing event or thought in their head. Studies show that this behavior is the number one predictor of depression. In my study, I found that men ruminate far less than women.

Why do women ruminate more than men? One explanation is that hormonal fluctuations, due to adolescence, pregnancy, childbirth, and menopause, drive some of these differences.

Another explanation is psychological: your default mode as a woman is to ruminate or think about your depressive feelings more than men.[3] But that doesn't mean you can't change that behavior.

The next time you find yourself overthinking by replaying a negative event, practice thought-stopping behavior:

1. **Yell "Stop!"** out loud to intentionally force yourself to shift your focus away from negative emotions.
2. **Change a Word:** Instead of saying "Yes, but . . ." say "Yes, and . . ." "Yes, but . . ." is often associated with a negative outlook. Practice positive reframing by thinking of positive things related to the situation. Using phrases like "Yes, and . . ." helps us consciously reframe situations. Scientists found that the more often we positively reframe situations, we can rewire our brain circuitry to shift toward more positive moods.[4]

Happiness and the Higher Power Agent

Another aspect of agency that influences happiness is whether you believe in a force that acts in the world and causes events to happen—that is, God. When something positive happens to you, you attribute that to a higher power. When something negative happens to you, you interpret it as a challenge for which God will give you the fortitude to endure and even overcome.

How would you answer these questions?

- How often do you go to religious service?

- Besides religious service, how often do you take part in other activities at a place of worship?
- Do you believe in a higher power who watches over you?
- Do you feel a deep sense of responsibility for reducing pain and suffering in the world?

Believe it or not, these questions can determine your mental health. Read over those questions again. The more strongly you feel about them, the more impact they can have on your happiness. That is what researchers at the University of Missouri found when they asked these questions of almost 160 people from different faiths: Buddhists, Muslims, Jews, Catholics, and Protestants, ranging from eighteen to eighty years old.[5]

The first two questions represent your views on what the researchers call "organizational religiousness." This measures how frequently you are involved in formal public religious events. The more often you go to religious services and take part in religious service, the more physically healthy you tend to be. One explanation for this has to do with lifestyle choices. If you are invested in your religious beliefs, then you are likely making choices that align with your religious beliefs, like less substance use and typically better dietary choices.

The next two questions represent your views on religious values and beliefs. Researchers call this a sense of "spiritual experiences." Your responses to these questions can determine your mental health (measured by how happy and peaceful you feel). This means that when you believe someone greater than you is watching over you during both good and bad times, you are more likely to feel happier and at peace.

The same researchers conducted another study and found

that not all spiritual experiences are the same when it comes to the effects that they have on mental health. *Negative spiritual belief* is the idea that if you don't do something right, God won't love you. It seems that 10 percent of us have this outlook.[6] Those who have this outlook feel abandoned or punished by a higher power when they have a health condition (like cancer or chronic pain). If you have that negative spiritual belief, you experience worse pain and are less happy than people who have a more positive spiritual outlook. If you are someone who believes that God loves you and forgives you despite your shortcomings, you will feel happier.

Here is what's interesting: Women are more likely to rely on support, like religion and God, to help them through tough times.

Truth:

Women seek emotional and spiritual support more often than men, which can improve their happiness.

In fact, they do so almost one third more than men, according to a survey conducted by Pew Research Center.[7] American women say religion is "very important" in their lives. They are also more likely than men to pray regularly and attend church services weekly. However, this gender gap in religion is not the same across different societies or religions. In sub-Sahara Africa, little difference exists between men and women when it comes to religious commitment in both Christian and Muslim faiths.

Why is there a gender gap in religion in the United States? Sociologists suggest that it has to do with our roles in the workforce.[8] Men traditionally work outside the home, while women traditionally work inside the home. As a result, women may turn to religion for social support. In fact, women often have more access to resources that offer support, like friendships and social networks.

Women who work full-time are often less religious than women who work inside the home. They also hold similar religious perspectives to men who work full-time outside the home. This pattern holds true across forty-seven countries: women in the workforce are typically less religious (measured by daily prayer, weekly service attendance, and how important religion is in their life) compared with women who don't work outside the home. In Scandinavian countries, where they have the highest rates of women working outside the home, women tend to be among the most secular. It is likely that working outside the home offers women equivalent levels of comfort and social support as religion does for women working inside the home.

Yet spirituality offers something distinct that boosts your happiness. It offers the reassurance that a higher power is watching over you, especially when you aren't able to control a situation (like a relationship, a health condition, or the loss of a job).

I saw this perspective on difficult times in a friend's social media post. This was their interpretation of a verse from the Bible (James 1:2–4).

1. Troubles lead to a test of faith.
2. When our faith is tested, our endurance grows.
3. We will one day reach a bullet-proof level of endurance.

God-mediated control is the idea that God works together with you to help you overcome challenges. Michael McCullough, a psychologist at the University of Miami, sheds light on this belief: "The mind really craves an explanation for the good and the bad, in terms of agency."[9] If your perspective is that challenges are part of a divine plan for your personal growth and development, then you are more likely to feel grateful when difficult situations arise in your life. This sense of gratitude acts as a buffer against the effects of stress.

To boost your happiness, keep in mind that your approach to religion matters. Focus on the experience rather than the checklist of attending religious events. Your perspective also matters. Adopt a positive spiritual belief, one based on a view of a loving God rather than a God who is out to punish you.

Happiness and Gratitude

Despite research that tells us about brain wiring and happiness, you may have heard that happiness is a choice. I have said it to others and even to myself many times. But how do you choose happiness if your brain is working against you? Gratitude. It changes your brain when it comes to happiness.

Neal Krause, a researcher from the University of Michigan, asked one thousand people about finances, depressed feelings, and gratitude. It turns out that having a sense of gratitude reduces depression by about 50 percent![10] Gratitude with religious or spiritual beliefs has a cascading effect:

- Taking part in religious events →
- The belief in God, a higher power in charge →
- Positive changes in gratitude →
- Increase in happiness

Why do we see this connection? Krause suggests that people who attend religious events regularly are more likely to feel grateful over time, compared with those who don't. In part, attending a religious service enhances the belief that God or a higher power is in control of events around you, which results in gratitude. And gratitude is a powerful way to buffer against real-life stresses.

Every morning I start my day with five minutes of gratitude. Some days it is directed toward someone greater than me, but other days, it is an utterance, words I say aloud to express what I am thankful for.

Dr. Michael McCullough from the University of Miami and his colleague found that a small action of gratitude can make a big impact on our mental health. They recruited two hundred people and divided them into these groups:

1. One group was asked to: "Think back over the past week and write down . . . up to five things in your life that you are grateful or thankful for."[11]

   Examples of gratitude expressions from the study include:

   - waking up this morning
   - the generosity of friends
   - to God for giving me determination
   - for wonderful parents
   - to the Rolling Stones

2. Another group was asked to "think back over today and . . . list up to five hassles that occurred in your life."[12]

   Examples of hassles from the study include:

111

- messy kitchen no one will clean
- finances depleting quickly
- stupid people driving
- doing a favor for friend who didn't appreciate it

Expressing gratitude results in feeling better about your life as a whole, as well as feeling more optimistic about the next week, compared to thinking about the hassles of the week.

Even a simple act of gratitude, like writing a letter of gratitude, changes the brain. A brain-scanning study found that expressing gratitude can train your brain to be more sensitive to being more grateful in the future. The researchers suggest that the more you practice gratitude, the more attuned you are to it, which results in happiness.[13] And these effects last! When the researchers brought the participants back in to the brain scanner months later, they still displayed the same brain activation patterns associated with gratitude three months later.

While it's true that your brain is wired uniquely to ruminate more, your brain can learn happiness by keeping it healthy, stop it from getting stuck, and practicing gratitude. In some ways, happiness *can* be your choice.

Summary: When it comes to happiness, women's brains are wired to ruminate more, which may influence one's sense of happiness. But simple habits can keep your brain happy.

Think Like a Girl

1. Keep your brain healthy—and happy.

- **Exercise:** This is one effective way to tackle your

brain's neurochemistry. For example, a randomized controlled study found that exercise was as effective as medication.[14] Why does exercise work? It boosts norepinephrine, which can in turn combat depression.

But it is often hard to be motivated, especially when you are struggling with mental health issues. So start with one simple action. "I'll wear running shoes today." Wearing running shoes can make you more likely to exercise than when you wear non-exercise shoes.

2. **Spirituality helps.**

- **Your approach to religion matters:** Focus on the experience rather than the checklist of attending religious events.

- **Perspective shift:** If you are religious or spiritual, examine your perspective for negative spiritual beliefs. Positive spiritual beliefs based on benevolence or love will support an overall sense of happiness.

3. **Agency matters.**

Instead of ruminating (overthinking), focus on what you can control. There are research-driven ways to change this default behavior.

- **Yell "stop":** The next time you find yourself overthinking by replaying a negative event, say "stop" aloud to force your focus away from the negative emotion.

- **Change a word:** Instead of saying "Yes, but . . ." say "Yes, and . . ." "Yes, but . . ." is often associated with a negative outlook. Practice positive reframing by thinking of positive things related to the situation.

- **Express thanks:** Gratitude is one way to change your brain when it comes to happiness. Having a belief that God or a higher power is in control of events around you results in gratitude, which can buffer against real-life stresses, like financial strain. Expressing gratitude by reflecting on five things you are grateful for in the past week or writing a letter thanking someone are some other ways to change the brain when it comes to happiness.

- **Bite a pencil:** This weird action has the power to trick your brain into being happy. It's called the facial feedback hypothesis, and its premise is that your actions can direct your emotions. It's the idea that the way in which you contract your muscles not only communicates what you are feeling to the people around you but also sends a message to your brain. Your facial expressions can change the way you feel. Smiling makes you happier; frowning makes you feel more negative emotion (like sadness or anger).

  So why does biting a pencil work? The action of biting the pencil forces your facial muscles into a smile. This fake smile uses the same muscles as a real one, signaling your brain that you are happy. According to almost 140 studies of more than eleven thousand people from around the world, facial expressions can interact with the conscious experience of emotion.[15] Our brain constantly monitors what our body is doing, and this can affect our emotions. If you sit in a slouched position, you tend to feel sad. If you cause your face to smile using a pencil, it tells your brain you are happy.

Get more quirky tips from my app, Brappy, available on both Google Play and Apple App stores.

Eight

The Generous Brain

Why Women Give

It started with a potato.

In December 2014 a curious thing happened on the internet. And it happened in quite an unremarkable way. It was a simple request. A request about an ordinary event. An event that some of us do quite often. Yet by some odd chance, this event ended up capturing the interest of millions of people.

> Basically I'm just making potato salad. I haven't decided what kind yet.

When Ohio-based Zack Brown sat down in front of his computer on a sunny July day and wrote that statement, he wasn't expecting the response he received. He was on the crowdfunding platform Kickstarter and asked for ten dollars to assist him in his project of making potato salad, admitting, "It might not be that good. It's my first potato salad."

His project started out as a gag. Brown and his friends were joking about having a potato-salad party to celebrate the Fourth of July, so he created the Kickstarter campaign to fund it. He was planning on only sending a preview link to his friends.[1]

A quick look at Google searches reveals that "potato salad" is most searched for the day before the Fourth of July.[2] So when Kickstarter verified Brown's information on July 3, it was almost too good of an opportunity to pass up. He set his campaign to go live and sent his friends a link to the real campaign. Thirty days later, Brown ended up with close to $56,000. For potato salad!

As the donations grew, Zack added to his promises. For example, twenty dollars won you the following:

- potato-salad themed haiku written by Zack
- your name carved into a potato that will be used in the potato salad
- a signed jar of mayonnaise
- the potato salad recipe
- hang out in the kitchen with Zack while he makes the potato salad
- choose a potato-salad-appropriate ingredient to add to the potato salad
- receive a bite of the potato salad
- a photo of Zack making the potato salad
- a thank-you posted to Zack's website
- Zack will say your name out loud while making the potato salad[3]

The grand prize for a $110 donation was called the Platinum Potato. The donor would receive the recipe book, the shirt and the hat along with a bite of the potato salad, a photo of Zack making the potato salad, a thank-you posted to his website, and a shout-out while he made the potato salad. Not a bad haul!

Potato Salad and You

As a woman, would you have given to Brown's potato salad fundraiser? How many times have you donated online? You may have not donated to a Kickstarter campaign. But you have probably donated to a friend's charity of choice on Facebook. Instead of asking for a birthday gift, Uncle Bob, whom you see only once a year, or your high school friend Kim asks you to join them in supporting the cause of a nonprofit organization. Causes can range from giving to a local school, to an arts project, to an ocean cleanup.

Digital altruism is a term that researchers have coined to describe acts that show concern for someone else's wellbeing using digital technology. These altruistic acts differ from in-person ones because they require little effort and are typically quick, like clicking on a link or watching an ad that results in a charity donation. Digital altruism is all around us, from online shopping, where a portion of the purchase price is donated to charity, to various gaming sites where correct answers lead to donations in community care, like water and medicine.

Crowdfunding is at the forefront of digital altruism. Although I have never set up a fundraiser on Kickstarter (yet!), I did contribute when a friend self-published her cookbook. My friend

Jessica, like me, is of Sri Lankan heritage, and her food pictures on Instagram brought me a sense of nostalgia and longing. They reminded me of many hours my mother and grandmother would spend in the kitchen and the delicacies that emerged. While I imagine my contribution to their culinary process to have been integral to the final dishes, in truth, I often did the easy tasks, like shell cardamoms, ground cinnamon, or deseed chilis. (The latter task was my least favorite; I would often rub my eyes, forgetting the potency of the chili on my fingers!)

Given that a big part of my childhood memories involve food, it was an easy decision to click on the donate button when Jessica sent her request to crowdfund her cookbook project. In exchange, I received a PDF copy of her cookbook, complete with mouthwatering illustrations, though I will admit that I was slightly envious of the donor who received the big prize: a dinner for two, prepared in person by Jessica.

Most donors are like you and me: we pledge small amounts toward a project. Zack Brown's potato salad fundraiser was no different, with about 70 percent of his backers pledging between one and four dollars. Fundraisers usually can't meet their target with these small donations alone. For Brown, the biggest funds came from just twelve people. Most of his donors, 75 percent or so, were men. This gender demographic is not much different from typical Kickstarter visitors, which, according to one report, are 75 percent male.[4]

Myth:

Women give more than men.

Self-report surveys show that women report being more generous than men, but these differences aren't consistent across studies. In some studies, women appear more generous. For example, single women are reported to give more to charities than single men. However, married people of both sexes give away a similar amount of money.[5]

A more systematic way to look at how men and women donate is when they are in the lab setting. This allows us to set up a microcosm of how you and I would give money to others. Other factors like social expectations, agreement with your partner, or even whether your donation is visible to the public can all be controlled in a lab setting. This approach lets researchers focus on one or two main factors without confusing the data.

The Giving Game

Play a game with me. Imagine you are in a large well-lit lecture hall. Although other people are around, they are some distance away. Other than a nod across the room, no one is interacting. I give you a number. This number is yours and only yours. Don't lose it. You will not be given a replacement number. You have to use it to collect your earnings at the end of the game.

Next I give you some tokens and pair you with another person in the lecture hall. Now you have some decisions to make. The tokens are worth different amounts depending on what you do with them. You will exchange them eight times, with the number of tokens you exchange going up along the way and the value per token going down as the number of tokens goes up. At the end of eight rounds, you can use your number to collect your earnings. There is only one player—you—and you have all the power to make the decisions. Here is how it works when you have fifty tokens.

Scenario 1: Generosity doubles the benefits for the other player.

- For tokens you keep for yourself, you receive ten cents for each token.
- For tokens you give away, the other player receives twenty cents for each token you pass on.
- You can keep them all, give them all away, or keep some and share some.

Scenario 2: Selfishness pays (triple!).

- For tokens you keep for yourself, you receive thirty cents for each token.
- For tokens you give away, the other player receives ten cents for each token you pass on.
- You can keep them all, give them all away, or keep some and share some.

This is called the dictator game. Social psychologists and economists use this "game" to understand whether a player will choose to share a cash prize with a stranger. There is no penalty for any of the decisions. The reward varies based on whether the player chooses to keep all the money or share it. The premise is that people will act out of a selfish drive to obtain the most amount of money, rather than opt to share a portion with a stranger.

Researchers at the University of Iowa and the University of Wisconsin put men and women into the dictator game to find out more about how and why we give.[6] The researchers found that contrary to what we might think, neither group is more generous than the other. Both groups gave the same amount of money to the stranger in their group.

Here is where differences emerge. Remember that the tokens are worth different values. Think of the trade-off between your own payoff and giving to the other player. This relative price of giving makes an impact on how we give. And it makes men and women behave differently.

What happens when the tokens are worth more money—when the payoff is greater for you to keep the token? Men, on average, increase the number of tokens they keep for themselves. Women show a different pattern when the payoff is greater for them: they decrease the proportion of tokens that they keep.

Truth: Women are equally as generous as men, but women are generous for more social reasons.

When the token has more value for the other player, women are more generous. They will give more than men. But when the tokens are cheaper for the other player, men give more.

Does this pattern bear out in the real world? Tipping in restaurants is one example that matches this data. A man's tip percentage is more responsive to the bill size than a woman's tip. As the bill size increases, men's tips decline at a faster rate than those of women. The magic number seems to hover around thirty dollars, where men tend to tip better than women for that amount or less. But above that, women are reported to tip better (percentagewise).[7]

Giving and Feelings

Why do you give? You give because you feel. By now you know that women are emotional creatures, and your feeling brain influences your decisions, relationships, happiness, and more.

Charities know this. That's why they have a picture of a single individual as the touchstone of their campaign.

You have probably seen the ad with the girl holding out her hand. It feels as if she is reaching out across the TV or computer screen to you. She tells you that a small donation, less than the price of a cup of coffee, will give clean water to her and her family for a month.

This is known as the *one person vs. big cause* approach. If someone tells you that fresh water is scarce in certain parts of the world and your donation is important, you probably won't believe them. This big cause is too overwhelming and makes your potential contribution feel like it will be just a drop in the bucket compared with the magnitude of the need.

A visual of a single individual, however, creates a connection between you, the giver, and the cause. When you look into that young girl's eyes, you know you can make a real difference for her. It grounds your donation to something tangible. And this connection intensifies the emotions you feel. The next time you pull into a coffee shop, you will probably also put aside something to give to this organization. You may even put a magnet of the girl's face on your fridge.

Truth:

Women give because they feel empathy.

To get to that point, we have to understand what is happening in the brain.

In a lab in California, twenty people are lying flat on their backs while inside a brain scanner.[8] They lie still and look at photos of people (six males and six females) and are asked to imitate their facial expressions of anger, fear, happiness, or sadness. The researchers are testing the power of mirror neurons.

Mirror neurons fire when you watch someone do an action. For example, when you see someone pick up a mug, the motor areas of your brain light up. The same thing happens with emotions. When you see a happy face, you may find yourself smiling too. And when you see someone who is angry, your brow furrows in response. It is for this reason that they are called the mind's mirror.

Mirror neurons explain a powerful social phenomenon, one that is thought to be the precursor for altruism. Mirror neurons help to explain empathy in the brain. Empathy starts with imitation, which begins shortly after birth. Babies begin imitating behavior, like moving their fingers, sticking out their tongues, and opening their mouth, when they are just a few weeks old.

We often think we are born with a sense of empathy, that it is a reflex like sucking and rooting behaviors. But we learn social interactions by observing and imitating others. These nascent social interactions and imitation games form the foundation for developing empathy.

Back to the lab in California. When the participants came out of the scanner, they played the dictator game. What do mirror neurons have to do with the dictator game and empathy? The researchers found that some people had supercharged mirror neurons. When they were asked to imitate facial expressions, they showed the strongest brain responses, especially in areas of the brain related to feelings (amygdala) and empathy. They were also more generous, giving away about 75 percent of their money in the game. The researchers called this the "mirroring impulse" because having to imitate other people's expressions activated their mirror neurons. And when their mirror neurons were firing strongly, they felt more empathy and connection and as a result were more likely to give away more of their winnings!

In contrast, the participants who showed the most brain activity in the front of the brain, the prefrontal cortex, were the least generous. On average they gave away only about 10 to 30 percent of the money. Why? This part of the frontal brain is responsible for controlling impulses and managing behavior. When you are busy thinking about the request for money, you are less likely to give. The prefrontal cortex is the responsible party: it functions as the one who vets decisions, sets a goal, and makes the plans to carry it out. It is not likely to let you give money away just because you *feel* something.

If you want to feel more generous, you need to dial down your prefrontal cortex and amp up your empathy. You may be one of those people with the supercharged mirror neurons! Even if not, you can develop your empathy and generosity. The quickest way to do that? Look at a photo and imitate the facial expressions you see. This simple action can stimulate your mirror neurons, making you more likely to act generously. You can also do this while having a conversation with someone. You may be someone who naturally "mirrors" the facial expressions of the person you are talking to. If not, you can train yourself to mirror their expressions by smiling when they smile and so on. Through practice, your empathy and generosity will grow.

Giving and a Sense of Belonging

So far we know that empathy is a key driver in acting generously. But men and women *feel* empathy for different reasons. As a result, we respond differently to giving. But how does empathy relate to the new wave of generosity: digital altruism?

In an effort to uncover our levels of magnanimity online, a graduate student, Heather, and I created a social media behavior scale. We wanted to understand how people interact online, from prosocial (helping) behaviors to negative behaviors, like starting arguments. We recruited participants from college campuses, the community, and of course social media sites to respond to questions about how connected they feel with people online, why they use social media platforms, and whether they demonstrate giving behaviors online. The first thing we did was to measure the participants' sense of altruism, with questions like, "It is my duty to help other people when they are unable to help themselves."

We also looked at their levels of empathy based on their online interactions. For example, we asked if they thought the way they treated people online would improve the day of the people who received the kind remarks. Would they interact with someone's post if they thought it affected their self-esteem? Or if it would make them smile?

Those types of prosocial behaviors were linked to a sense of belonging and community. But, as it turns out, a sense of empathy or concern for how other people feel online wasn't a significant driving force when it comes to feeling altruistic. This pattern was true both for the men and women in my study.

Our data show us that there are different motivations for men and women and how they feel they should help others. For women, the more socially connected they feel, the more likely they are to act in an altruistic way. A sense of belonging, represented by a desire to make friends online, made the women in my study feel more connected. When women feel a sense of belonging, they have a heightened sense of empathy. And as a result, they are more likely to act generously.

For the men, it was a different story. They are more motivated by a need to protect. I call it the "be a hero" motivation. They responded strongly to statements like the following:

- I feel obligated to respond when I see someone is being bullied on social media.
- I worry about what will happen if I don't intervene when someone is being bullied on social media.
- I feel I must say something positive when I see a rude comment on someone's status.

This set of statements reflects our need to protect, to be a hero. The more strongly a guy feels that he has to defend someone, the more likely he is to act generously and altruistically.

Costly Signaling Theory

Costly signaling theory refers to behaviors that appear extravagant and even wasteful. In other words, they don't seem to have a direct benefit or an immediate purpose. Instead, they serve as a signal to convey certain information about the person. According to this theory, a man's "saving the day" approach is a way to advertise desirable personal traits, which makes it more likely for him to attract a suitable mate. So when a guy defends someone online or calls out a bully on social media, it is a sign that he is advertising his positive qualities.

To boost your generosity, find your tribe. When you feel surrounded and supported by a community (even an online community), you are more likely to act in a generous manner—and not only financially. That might mean you're more willing to share your time to help someone. Or it might mean you're more willing to share your expertise with a friend who needs help.

Summary: Women typically give money away when the payoff is greater for the recipient. Women also give because we feel empathy and when we have a sense of belonging.

Think Like a Girl

If you want to feel more generous, dial down your prefrontal cortex and amp up your empathy. You may be wondering why or when you might need to feel more generous. If you're a parent or caregiver, many situations arise when you have to prioritize someone else's needs over your own. Although we often hear how important it is to take "me time" (and it is), that is not always possible when you have little ones tugging at you, needing your attention and your energy. In moments like those, here are some ways you can boost your empathy.

1. **Imitate me!**

   Mirror neurons are neurons in your brain that fire when you watch someone do an action. The same thing happens with emotions. Mirror neurons help us develop empathy. If you want to be more generous, look at someone and try to imitate their facial expressions. This activates your mirror neurons, which boosts empathy.

2. **Find your tribe.**

   Make friends and be part of a community, even if online. Making friends online results in a sense of belonging, which can lead to altruism.

Part Five

The Leader Brain

Nine

The Empathy Brain

Redefining Empathy in the Workplace

Elena Gomez stared across the table at her boss. She blinked quickly. She couldn't believe what she was hearing. She had worked so hard to get to this point.

On a management team of mostly men, Gomez is the chief financial officer (CFO) of Zendesk. Zendesk is a Silicon Valley company that builds software to elevate customer relationships. Gomez is their first female CFO. Her credentials have earned her a seat at the table. As a graduate of the University of California-Berkeley, she previously worked at Charles Schwab and Visa.

Despite her impressive résumé and string of accomplishments, she had been summoned. Her boss was reprimanding her. She had missed the mark. "It's more important to be respected than to be liked," he said to her. On a spectrum between "like" and "respect," he explained, she was so well liked that she needed to pivot her focus beyond this value.

Gomez echoes that phrase during her interview with me. "Don't worry about being liked, but worry about being respected," she says. I type furiously as she talks. Behind her is a wall of books. She is dressed in black and is immaculately groomed, even when working from home. I tuck a stray hair behind my ear and find myself squaring my shoulders to sit up straighter. She exudes confidence and magnetism, even across a computer screen.

"I often have to share bad news. I have learned over time to worry about being respected and holding my ground. It is the same when giving feedback to an employee. The bias is that you want to be liked. And it is an implied feeling: if you give someone feedback, they will no longer like you." For Gomez, her conversation with her boss shifted her thinking. She realized that doing her job sometimes means she has to move away from focusing on how someone is feeling and whether they will like her.

Myth:

Women need to be more empathetic in the workplace.

According to Kim Scott, a business coach, "We're conditioned from an early age to avoid hurting people's feelings. It's not a bad impulse to protect people's feelings, but it's a short-lived protection. You need to rise above your empathy and realize that it's your own feelings you are protecting, not theirs."[1]

I share this idea with Gomez. "Hmm, interesting," she responds. I go on.

Ruinous empathy is a phrase used to characterize what happens when you care too much. Ruinous empathy holds people back from negotiating for themselves. "Yes, I've seen that in my workplace. Especially with junior members," Gomez replies.

Empathy can also be a poor moral guide. Yes, you read that correctly. Although empathy often helps us do what's right, it can also motivate us to do what's wrong.

Let me tell you a story.

There is a charity called the Quality Life Foundation. This foundation works hard to make the final years of terminally ill children as comfortable as possible. Enter Sheri Summers, a brave and bright ten-year-old. Little Sheri has a muscle-paralyzing disease known as *myasthenia gravis.* Symptoms of this autoimmune disease include muscle weakness, such as drooping eyelids, lopsided facial muscles, and even trouble walking. For Sheri, simple things like opening a door or reading were extremely challenging. She was on a waiting list for extremely expensive medication. The medication wouldn't lengthen her life, but it would improve the quality of it. But as with most illness, the list was long, and Sheri's prospects did not look good.

There was another list: The immediate help list. If Sheri could make it on this list, then the Quality Life Foundation would fund this expensive medication. But other children were on the waiting list ahead of Sheri. They too had terminal illnesses and could benefit from support from the Quality Life Foundation. Severity of their condition and time left to live typically determine the decisions about which children get moved from the waiting list to the immediate help list.

Here is where you come in. You have been given the unexpected opportunity to move Sheri to the immediate help list. You could literally and dramatically change the quality of her life. You have met Sheri. Her little voice talking about how each daily activity is a battle rings in your ears. Maybe you have a child around the same age as Sheri. You can't help but wonder what it would be like if your child experienced the same struggles. Surely you would like to find a way to make their life more comfortable.

Read the story again. This time, try to take an objective perspective. Remain detached as you make your decision. And remember, if you choose to move Sheri, then other children who are on the waiting list who may have greater needs or shorter life expectancy will have to wait longer.

That is exactly what psychologist Daniel Batson and his colleagues asked participants to do. When asked to think of Sheri as they read her story, Batson found that almost 75 percent of people were willing to move her to the immediate help list.[2] They were so involved in Sheri's story that they overlooked the other children who had greater needs than she did.

Compare that with the people who were asked to take an objective perspective as they heard Sheri's story. Only a third of them were willing to let Sheri skip the line and benefit from the Quality Life Foundation.[3]

Empathy can create tunnel vision. You are so focused on someone else's pain that you want to take action, even at the expense of others. Although Sheri's story is fictional, created purely for research purposes, it is an echo of real life. Another psychologist, Paul Bloom, shows how empathy leads to inefficient decisions when Make-A-Wish spends thousands of dollars so that a terminally ill child can live out a dream (like being Batman), while the money could have been used to support multiple children instead.[4]

On a small scale, that is what Gomez was doing: focusing on the discomfort that a critique would cause. So she pulled back. She didn't want to be the person delivering the bad news. No one likes that messenger. But focusing on not wanting to hurt someone's feelings can result in employees not knowing how to improve their work and become better team players. Gomez is recalibrating. "If I want to be liked, I might give in even though it is not the best outcome," she says to me. "Now I say what I need. I've learned how to negotiate better, and I hope to garner respect for holding my ground."[5]

Are Women Hardwired for Empathy?

Was Gomez at a disadvantage? Are women hardwired to feel more empathic? British psychologist Simon Baron-Cohen wanted to explore this idea more. So with his team of researchers, he looked at a genetic sampling of over forty-five thousand people, with a roughly even split of males and females.[6]

This old debate pops up for most behavioral issues. Do you blame your parents for bad genes, or do you blame your parents for bad parenting? I'm joking of course. But here is the question: Is empathy heritable? The researchers found three pieces of evidence that address this question.

1. There was no difference in heritability between males and females. In other words, women aren't born more empathetic then men.
2. There was a high genetic correlation between the males and the females. This means that the genetic architecture of empathy in males and females was highly similar.
3. The link between the genetic architecture of empathy and self-reported empathy was the same between men and women. Self-reported empathy was measured with

Truth:

Women are not born with more empathy than men, but they are socially rewarded for their empathy.

questions like: "I can easily tell if someone else wants to enter a conversation" or "I find it difficult to explain to others things that I understand easily, when they don't understand it the first time."[7]

However, that's just the beginning of the story on empathy. While men and women are generally born with a similar capacity for empathy, as girls grow into women and their hormonal development diverges from that of boys, their empathic skills change as well.

Empathy: What Do You See?

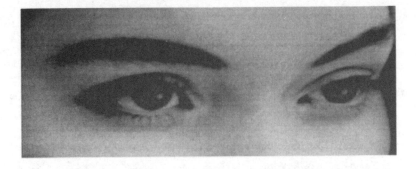

Look into those eyes above. What do you see?

Choose one word that best describes what you think the person is thinking or feeling. The word you choose may seem automatic, as if by instinct. You may not know why you chose it.

Now choose a word from this list to describe what you think the person is thinking or feeling:

reflective

aghast

irritated

impatient

According to Baron-Cohen, women are more likely to guess that those eyes look reflective. He developed the Eyes Test to measure social cognition in adults, or how well you can put yourself in another person's mind and "tune in to what they are feeling"[8] just by looking at their eyes. In his research lab, he asked participants to select one of four emotions that best described twenty-five pairs of eyes similar to the one at the beginning of this chapter. Baron-Cohen found that women answer on average twenty-one correct; men almost 20 percent less.[9] Women are better than men at detecting someone's emotions just from looking at their eyes.

The ability to read other people's emotions is critical to survival. When you read happiness in someone's eyes, you are more likely to approach them. When you read anger in someone's eyes, you may want to take cover!

I show Gomez these eyes. What does she see? I am curious.

"Cautious. Reflective," she says without missing a beat.

What helps you detect the emotion behind those eyes? All it takes is a little dose of estrogen, which women have more of than men. Here is something interesting: When men were given a hormone concoction of estrogen, their responses to the Eyes Test changed. Their focus switched. Previously, they detected dominance in the eyes. They looked at the brows. They looked at whether the eyes were furrowed. They weren't tuned in to the emotions to the same extent as the women were. With the "exogenous dose" (which means externally) of estrogen, the men showed an increase in their attention to the emotional states of others.

New research suggests that the reason for why women express empathy more than men is nuanced and relies on an interplay between hormones and the environment. Nurture also plays a powerful role in shaping the brain. And it starts in infancy.

Empathy: Add a Little Nurture

A soft, flannel blanket lies on the ground. Four toys and one baby book—the kind that babies like to chew—are scattered close by. The scene sounds like it could be a nursery or daycare. But it is a research lab.

Truth:

Women can express more empathy and read others' emotions better than men because of estrogen levels that change throughout the lifespan.

The mother lays her baby on the blanket—just the two of them are in the room. She coos softly, "Mommy loves her little bunny." She wiggles his toes. The baby coos back. Her phone buzzes. She briefly looks at it. Her baby kicks his feet in the air. "Mommy's here," she chirps, putting away her phone. She picks up a toy. "Look at this puppy. Puppy says hello." She bops the toy puppy gently on her baby's nose. He giggles and reaches out for it. She hides the toy behind her back. "Where did puppy go?" Her baby's eyes widen. "Here is puppy," she says, bopping the toy on her baby's nose again. They play their game a little longer. Five minutes later, the cameras are turned off. The mother and baby leave the room.

This mother was one of over one hundred women and babies who participated in a study to find out how empathy is cultivated.[10] The mothers were in their thirties, and their babies were five months old. They returned for a second session in the lab when the baby was eighteen months old. While the mother was busy playing with her infant, the researchers were busy recording their interactions. They watched the videos to see how often she talked to her baby, how much attention she gave to her baby, and whether she reached out to her baby. The researchers also watched the babies. Did they laugh when their mother played with them? How was their mood? Did they smile a lot?

A mother's involvement when she is playing with her child sends a powerful signal. And that signal can be measured from their spit. Saliva samples were collected both from the mother and her baby, and then again a year later when they came back to the lab.

Child: Infancy represents a sensitive time period in development, where the brain regions related to oxytocin development are dynamic and sensitive to the social environment. When a mother is highly involved in playtime with her baby, this results in changes in the oxytocin receptor gene in her baby.

Mother: No changes occur in the oxytocin receptor gene when she plays with her child. This means that her genetic levels are stable in adulthood.

Nurture, in the form of your social environment during infancy, can make a difference when it comes to empathy. Men and women both benefit from early nurturing interactions with their mother. After all, empathy is a learned skill.

If you find yourself needing to turn *up* the volume on your empathy levels, then take a page from research. Practice looking people directly in the eyes and see if you can read their emotions. Follow this up by asking them directly, "How are you feeling?"

Another tact is to get on social media. My research shows that social media use can develop greater empathy skills in women.[11] People who spend more time sending messages and commenting on social media are more empathic. Take a moment to practice and experience empathy by connecting with someone on social media by sending them a message and engaging with them.

Empathy Redefined

So what do we do with empathy in the workplace? Empathy in the workplace is a little like the Goldilocks effect. Too much can be counterproductive, and too little can result in poor management. Just right is what you need. A recent survey of almost seven thousand managers across thirty-eight countries found a positive link between empathy and job performance.[12] The truth is that you can have empathy and gain respect in the workplace if you strike the right balance.

Truth:

The truth is that you can have empathy and gain respect in the workplace if you strike the right balance.

If you find yourself needing to turn *down* the volume on your empathy levels, rethink your priorities. If you shift your focus to the end goal instead of trying to spare someone else's feelings, it will be easier to avoid "ruinous empathy."

In truth, empathy isn't about being

liked or being a people pleaser. It isn't about being a pushover. Instead, empathy is the ability to understand others and the impact your actions have on them.

This is something Chloe Hakim-Moore understands very well. As a child, she split her time between Trinidad and the United States. When I talk to her, she shares how she grew up with cousins who were ethnically and racially diverse. Her exposure to different groups has helped her learn to see things from other people's perspectives.

She has taken this skill and applied it to her passion as the director of NEXT Memphis, which focuses on early childhood education. Moore is putting into practice a key principle in developing empathy in the workplace: she listens. A lot. And it helps her develop *perspective taking*: the ability to consider someone else's viewpoint. Social psychologists find that this skill matters.

Naturally, people categorize themselves into groups. They may use culture or ethnicity or interests to identify themselves with others in an in-group. This is known as *social identity theory*. You create your identity based on social dimensions that you value. The benefit of this approach is that you associate yourself with a group of similar people. The drawback, of course, is that if you aren't part of a particular in-group, understanding where they are coming from can be difficult.

Perspective taking requires you to think and feel what it would be like to be part of an out-group (a group that you don't view as similar to you). Before NEXT Memphis, Moore worked with refugees and immigrant populations. Working with them and growing up with a mother from Trinidad helped her develop her perspective-taking skills. Moore's efforts have placed her as one of the recipients of *Forbes*'s 30 under 30 (in 2018), a list that

Forbes says is "harder to get into than America's two most selective colleges, Stanford and Harvard University."[13]

One of the most effective ways to take someone else's perspective is to listen. Psychologists call this active listening. Here are some ways to do that:

- Shift the focus from your thoughts to what they are saying.
- Don't feel the need to fill conversation gaps with questions. Sometimes silence is their way to think through what they want to share.
- Repeat or paraphrase what they have just said ("It sounds like you are saying . . . ?"). One study found that this simple conversation tool builds closeness between the speaker and the listener.[14]

Another study looked at people who spent time intentionally adopting someone else's perspective for thirty minutes a day over three months. They found that this activity resulted in higher levels of perspective taking and structural changes in the brain areas associated with what the authors refer to as "feeling states."[15]

Gomez also puts this idea of perspective taking into practice. When I ask her what drives her decision-making process in the workplace, she replies, "As a leader you have to have high emotional intelligence. If I dominate a conversation, you will leave with a feeling that you didn't get what you want out of it, even if you don't tell me. I've learned that over time, I need to meet my colleague where they are."

Through her years of experience, Gomez understands the double-edged sword of empathy in the workplace: too much empathy and you can lose sight of the bigger goal because you are focused on the emotions of the individual; too little empathy and you miss the connection that you can build with your team. The tips in this chapter provide you with concrete ways to turn up or down your empathy so you can manage it and use it effectively.

Summary: Women may express more empathy in the workplace because they've been socialized toward this value, but it can be counterproductive. Too much empathy can create tunnel vision where you are so focused on feeling someone else's pain that you take action even at the expense of others. Empathy is not about being a pushover or people-pleasing. It is the ability to understand the impact your actions have on others.

Women aren't born more empathetic than men, but we are better at expressing it and detecting others' emotions. It's a dynamic and nuanced interaction between nature and nurture.

Think Like a Girl

Change your priority if empathy is hindering your job. Shift your focus to the end goal instead of someone else's feelings to avoid "ruinous empathy." Do a gut check: Are you modifying your behavior out of the driving desire to be liked, or are you practicing empathy as an authentic expression of who you are?

However, empathy takes practice. It's a skill we have to learn. Here are tips to develop it:

1. **Look into their eyes.**

    Practice looking people directly in the eyes and see if you can read their emotions. Follow this up by asking them directly, "How are you feeling?"

2. **Use active listening to take someone else's perspective:**
   - Shift the focus from your thoughts to what they are saying.
   - Don't feel the need to fill conversation gaps with questions. Sometimes silence is their way to think through what they want to share.
   - Repeat or paraphrase what they have just said ("It sounds like you are saying . . . ?").

3. **Flex your empathy muscles on social media.**

   In my TEDx Talk, I share my research on how social media can encourage empathy.[16] When we take time to engage on social media, intentionally acknowledging the individuals behind the avatars, we are able to practice and experience empathy.

Ten

The Leader Brain

*Busting the Myth That Women Need to
Lead like Men to Be Successful*

"Women need to interrupt. As the only woman in the room, I was often ignored. But I have a strong voice."

I was two rows away from Madeleine Albright, the first female Secretary of State and the highest-ranking woman in the history of the US government at that time. I looked over at my friend Christine Hoene and grinned in disbelief. Like every other person in the room, I was mesmerized. I couldn't believe I was listening to Albright talk. Story after story made the hour fly by! She talked about how she intentionally selected brooches to communicate a particular message as she met with a world leader, like the hear-no-evil, see-no-evil, speak-no evil monkeys when she met with Putin during their conflict with Chechnya and a snake pin when she met with Saddam Hussein after he had invaded Kuwait.

Albright was funny, entertaining, and even a little self-deprecating. But not when it came to her advice to women. "I say to my students, 'Don't raise your hand in my class. Interrupt,'" she said. "My class is a bit of a zoo," she added with a laugh. That stuck with me, especially as I had recently finished a project on female leaders and was curious to find out how perceptions of leadership impact mental health (more on that later).

Myth:

Women have to act like men to be effective leaders.

"Take my advice, Belinda: You'll never get to the top in this business if you spend all your time worrying about feelings. You've just got to sell, sell, sell."[1] That was the advice given to female executive Belinda Parmar, as shared to British newspaper the *Guardian*.

"Sound like a Gordon Ghekko parody? Sadly, this priceless nugget of wisdom came courtesy of my middle-management boss about a decade ago. Following his lead, I wondered if I was too caring to do my job well. I took to wearing black power-suits in an attempt to emulate hard-nosed businessmen. I became a carbon-copy caricature of a business executive in an attempt to mould myself into my image of what the board of directors might appreciate."[2]

Parmar's story is not unique. As I wrote this chapter, I came across story after story of women sharing how they dressed like men, walked like men, and used phrases that sounded more "masculine" to get ahead in the workplace. In every instance, the women said they wished they felt more comfortable leading in a way that felt natural to them. Some of their comments include: "They are far more task-oriented. . . . I have difficulty because I am not at all that way."

As a female academic, I know the feeling too. I am used to going to conferences that are predominantly male. Despite being the top-ranked researcher at my university, I was told (by a male colleague) that I "wasn't ready" for a promotion. Thankfully, I didn't agree, applied for the promotion, and got it.

Writing this chapter was particularly interesting for me. How can we change the myths that we as women believe about leadership? Are there things we hold on to that hold us back in the workplace?

Narcissism and Confidence

Numerous studies have documented the prioritization of masculine traits in leadership positions, traits like dominance, competitiveness, and narcissism. But does possessing these traits mean you are a successful leader?

While it is easy for us to label traits like narcissism as "good" or "bad," this trait can be positive and either "adaptive" or "maladaptive," depending on the situation. For example, studies show that people who score high in narcissism tend to take control of leaderless groups. Even trained observers saw narcissistic people as the natural leaders and would be more likely to hire them for managerial positions.[3] In those cases, the narcissism is adaptive, or positive.

However, for women, I found a unique pattern between narcissism and leadership styles in female leaders: high levels of narcissism are associated with a passive/avoidant style of leadership, which leads to stress and burnout.

When women leaders adopt narcissistic traits that seem more

"masculine," like always being right and needing to be the center of attention, it backfires! You end up using a passive leadership style that leaves you feeling ineffective and stressed as a result, thus maladaptive, or negative. Here's why: Narcissists seek out leadership roles because they like the power. They like being in charge, but they don't necessarily make good leaders who can build a team, make decisions for the greater good, or put aside self-interest to accomplish a bigger goal.

Another reason narcissism doesn't pay off for women is because you end up being judged more harshly than men. One Dutch study reported that women who display narcissistic traits are perceived as ineffective leaders.[4] But interestingly, this is true only when male subordinates evaluate female leaders. Female subordinates did not evaluate their female leaders as less effective even if they displayed narcissistic traits. And while it may not seem fair, men get a free pass when it comes to narcissism, from both male and female subordinates.

If women leaders should steer clear of adopting narcissistic traits in the workplace, what should they do instead? The antidote to narcissism is confidence. Yet women are notorious for not displaying confidence. In many studies, men typically overestimate their abilities and performance, while women underestimate both. Yet objective evaluations of both men and women's performances reveal that they don't differ in quality.[5]

An often-quoted, real-world example comes from Hewlett-Packard. They reviewed personnel records to learn more about why more women weren't in top management positions. They discovered that men applied for a more senior role if they thought they could meet 60 percent of the job requirements. In contrast, women would apply only if they believed they could meet 100 percent of the job qualifications.[6] Feeling confident only when you have a sense of 100 percent competency is tough! No wonder more women didn't apply for senior roles.

Truth:

Women are often less confident in the workplace, despite being equally competent.

This lack of confidence, despite our abilities, is prevalent. I provide consulting for a media company in New York City. As part of my consultancy, I developed and carried out research on a few hundred women in the workplace. Almost half of them said that they frequently feel a sense of imposter syndrome in the workplace. These women were also 25 percent more likely to experience stress and lower levels of job satisfaction as a result of this lack of confidence.

If you are reading this and it is resonating, maybe it is time to reevaluate your level of confidence in the workplace. Albright was on to something. You do need to interrupt. Not because you want to be the center of attention or because you think you are right but because you are confident in your voice. Because you recognize your accomplishments. Because you realize you do bring something to the table.

Christine Hoene knows this. Christine is the founder and CEO of LifeSafe Services. She grew the company from a single state business to a nationwide business, specializing in providing businesses with safety training (like CPR) and life-saving devices, like defibrillators. Her mission is to make sure that employees are prepared in an emergency.

I met Christine some years ago when I wandered into an aerial studio, mistakenly thinking I was signing up for a yoga class. Christine was the owner and had recently started the studio. We bonded over our love-hate relationship with the trapeze and the shared feeling of accomplishment when learning a new trick on the bar.

A cause that is close to Christine's heart relates to muscular dystrophy. One organization brought Christine in as a consultant to increase awareness and education. Her idea was to create a dance app to get people moving. The board wasn't convinced. But Christine knew it was the right idea for this group. At the age of forty-nine, she was diagnosed with FSH muscular dystrophy, a genetic disorder, and was told she would be using a walker within four or five years. That was almost ten years ago. Since her diagnosis, Christine has gone ice climbing, learned how to kite surf and mountain bike, and is one of the strongest people in aerial I know!

At that moment in the boardroom, she had to interrupt to make her voice heard. She pushed her idea. And it paid off! The app, the Live Dance Challenge, was a success and created a huge wave of awareness for the organization and what they were doing to support people with muscular difficulties. For Christine, each time she sees her success in one area, it fuels her confidence to try something new.

What is something that you have overcome that gives you confidence in who you are and what you can accomplish? The next time you find yourself second-guessing your abilities, stop to think about a specific event when you were successful. Then be confident in your approach and speak up. Here are some other tips to help build your confidence.

- **Power pose!** If you have an interview or presentation that is causing you to lose your confidence, practice a power pose. Stand with your hands on your hips, feet hip-width apart, like Superman or Wonder Woman, for two minutes.

Harvard University researchers found that this simple action can decrease cortisol (stress) by up to 25 percent.[7] Research demonstrates that people are more likely to follow those who display confidence, so get power posing!

- **Right side up.** If you are a right-hander, use your right hand when you are communicating an important statement to your team, a friend, or your significant other. Why does this work? Researchers from Stanford University found that right-handers tend to associate right-handed gestures with positive ideas and leftward gestures with negative ideas. The opposite pattern is found if you are a left-hander: these individuals are more likely than right-handers to associate left with positive ideas.[8] When you communicate with a right-handed person using your right hand, they will be more likely to view your ideas positively.

Style of Your Leadership

Now that you know how to display your confidence, let's find out what leadership traits you need to be a successful leader. My research students Chalow and Sam and I recruited almost four hundred people and asked them to identify their leadership style. Look at these styles and pick out yours:

Transformational Leadership

- I reexamine critical assumptions to question whether they are appropriate.
- I help others to develop.

Transactional Leadership

- I make clear what one can expect to receive when performance goals are achieved.
- I keep track of all mistakes.

Passive/Avoidant Leadership

- I wait for things to go wrong before taking action.
- I avoid making decisions.

Which pair of statements best reflects your leadership style?

Transformational leaders are described as inspirational, intellectually stimulating, and charismatic. A key characteristic of a transformational leader is his or her interest in working with people to achieve an outcome. They use social skills and emotional intelligence to motivate their team into action.

Transactional leaders focus on the task at hand and ensure that the needs of their associates are met. They focus on fairly compensating their workers based on the quality of their work. They actively set standards and often watch for mistakes. They don't act until the mistakes have occurred.

Passive/Avoidant leaders avoid action until mistakes can no longer be ignored. In some cases, they may avoid leadership altogether.

As with most topics, there are multiple theories, and leadership style is no exception. You may have heard of other leadership styles, like authoritative, delegative, and so on. The leadership styles I discuss in this chapter were chosen because they are some of the most commonly used in the workplace.

Leadership style matters. Here is what I found from my study. When women are passive/avoidant leaders, they are more likely to experience stress and burnout. Interestingly, it's not the same for male leaders. It seems counterintuitive, but not leading leads to more stress and burnout if you are a woman. In other words, doing nothing as a leader is bad for your mental health. There is no benefit in taking on "masculine" leadership traits. Often it will not feel natural. And worst-case scenario, you are perceived as an ineffective leader.

In contrast, women who adopt a more relationship-driven leadership style (transformational leader) are less likely to experience stress. This relationship-driven approach is often a more natural approach because of the social dynamics and focus on developing connections.

Leadership styles aren't about being masculine or feminine. They are about knowing which approach to use and when to use them. Psychologists agree that leadership styles aren't like personality traits: you aren't born with them, and they aren't fixed. A good leader knows when to be a transformational leader and when to be a transactional leader. After all, competitiveness is self-defeating in environments where cooperation is needed.

This is something Christine Hoene knows and practices as a leader. She understood early on that despite her ambition and her skill set, there were times when her board wouldn't listen to her simply because she was a woman. Christine describes one occasion when she and her then-husband,

Truth:

The best leadership style is one that adapts to the situation at hand and the needs of the team and company.

Patrick, had acquired and merged with another company. As they walked into the boardroom, Ken, one of the top team leaders, immediately looked at Patrick for leadership direction. It wasn't long before Patrick and Ken's leadership styles clashed.

When Christine had to step in, she decided to use a more transformative approach. She would go out of her way to solicit Ken's feedback on decisions. She praised her team frequently. And she saw dividends with this approach. It wasn't long before Ken was praising her leadership in front of the other board members. During a recent and controversial decision where the board was split, Ken spoke up and urged the members to listen to Christine's perspective on the issue.

What do you bring to the table as a leader? Ask yourself this question. The answer will likely reveal your natural leadership style. This chapter isn't here to give you a blueprint. It's here to affirm you. As my friend Christine did, you are probably already following your instincts and adopting the best approach for your team. But remember that your leadership style is not fixed. You aren't born with it. The best leaders are the ones who can adapt their style to the situation.

Summary: Women are less confident in the workplace, despite being equally competent. The best leadership style is neither masculine nor feminine but about knowing which styles to use and when to use them.

Think Like a Girl

1. Stay away from the passive/avoidant leadership style.
This approach can lead to stress and burnout.

2. **Boost and display your confidence.**
   - Avoid second-guessing your decisions.
   - Focus on your success.
   - Practice your power pose.
   - Use your right hand when you communicate an important statement to your team, a friend, or your significant other.

Just the Beginning

We have reached the final pages together, which brings me to the book's conclusion. However, I hope you think of this book as more of a beginning. The beginning of understanding why you do what you do. The beginning of learning your strengths as a woman and how to use them.

Myths spring up as part of a culture, especially when it comes to what a woman can and cannot do, what's considered "normal," and what's considered off-script. These myths represent a social perspective. I grew up in Malaysia, moved to the US when I was a young girl, and lived in Central America and the UK as an adult before moving back to the US. I heard many different myths about what I could do or shouldn't do as a woman.

While myths can be important, I wanted to know the truth beyond the myths. What does your brain say you can do?

This book represents my search. It has been germinating in my head for over three years. In part, I wrote it because I wanted answers for myself.

But I also want to share these answers. With my students in my psychology classes who want to change the status quo and have great ideas for a different future. With my bright-eyed young clients who want to know that their tomorrow could be different from today. With you, the reader, who has come on this journey with me.

Through these pages, I hope I was able to pull back the curtain so that you could see how remarkable your brain is and understand a little more about what gives you a unique strength—in decision-making, in leadership, in love, and more. I also hope you learned a few tips to maximize that strength and think like a girl.

Notes

Preface

1. Cathy Benko and Bill Pelster, "How Women Decide," *Harvard Business Review*, September 2013, https://hbr.org/2013/09/how -women-decide.https://hbr.org/2013/09/how-women-decide.
2. Benko and Pelster, "How Women Decide."
3. Joyce Ehrlinger and David Dunning, "Attitudes and Social Cognition: How Chronic Self-Views Influence (and Potentially Mislead) Estimates of Performance," *Journal of Personality and Social Psychology* 84, no. 1 (2003): 5–17, https://pdfs.semanticscholar .org/1f54/81ffac7c9495782c423b3de8034d8d2acba5.pdf.
4. Tara Sophia Mohr, "Why Women Don't Apply for Jobs Unless They're 100% Qualified," *Harvard Business Review*, August 25, 2014, https://hbr.org/2014/08/why-women-dont-apply-for-jobs -unless-theyre-100-qualified.

Chapter 1: The Stressed Brain

1. Ajay, "'You Stole a Point from Me, You're a Thief Too': Naomi Osaka Wins Serena Williams in US Open Final as She Slams Umpire I'm Not a Cheater," *Sports Tribunal*, September 9, 2018, https://sportstribunal.com/you-stole-a-point-from-me-youre-a -thief-too-naomi-osaka-wins-serena-williams-in-us-open-final -as-she-slams-umpire/.

2. "Serena Williams Goes Off on Umpire! Accuses Him of Sexism! Full Exchange," Raf Productions, September 8, 2018, YouTube video, 3:09, https://www.youtube.com/watch?v=GLcf9YqL8Ek.

3. Ted Osborn, "US Open Umpire Did the Right Thing, Serena Williams Just Had a Temper Tantrum," *South China Morning Post*, September 16, 2018, https://www.scmp.com/comment /letters/article/2164265/us-open-umpire-did-right-thing-serena -williams-just-had-temper.

4. Simeon Gholam, "Andy Murray Shows Off His Football Skills (with a Tennis Ball!) as He Trains Ahead of Wimbledon Quarter-Final Clash," *Daily Mail*, July 7, 2015, https://www.dailymail.co.uk/sport /tennis/article-3152344/Andy-Murray-shows-football-skills-tennis -ball-trains-ahead-Wimbledon-quarter-final-clash.html.

5. "Serena Williams Accuses Umpire of Sexism and Vows to 'Fight for Women,'" *Guardian*, September 9, 2018, https://www.theguardian .com/sport/2018/sep/09/serena-williams-accuses-officials-of-sexism -and-vows-to-fight-for-women.

6. Kaelen Jones, "Serena Williams Argues With Umpire, Receives One-Game Penalty During U.S. Open Loss," *Sports Illustrated*, September 8, 2018, https://www.si.com/tennis/2018/09/08/serena -williams-us-open-umpire-i-dont-cheat-win-id-rather-lose -naomi-osaka.

7. "An Issue Whose Time Has Come: Sex/Gender Influences on Nervous System Function," *Journal of Neuroscience Research* 95, no. 1–2 (January/February 2017), https://onlinelibrary.wiley.com /toc/10974547/2017/95/1-2.

8. Amitai Shenhav and Joshua D. Green, "Moral Judgments Recruit Domain-General Valuation Mechanisms to Integrate Representations of Probability and Magnitude," *Neuron* 67 (August 26, 2010): 667–77, https://static1.squarespace.com/static /54763f79e4b0c4e55ffb000c/t/594d7f42cd0f68696be4db60/14982 51082966/moral-judgments-recruit-domain-general-valuation -mechanisms-to-integrate-representations-of-probability-and -magnitude.pdf.

9. Liz Belilovskaya, "In Search of Morality: An Interview with Dr. Joshua Greene," *Brain World*, November 2, 2019, https://brain worldmagazine.com/in-search-of-morality-an-interview-with -joshua-greene/2/.

10. Manuella Fumagalli et al., "Brain Switches Utilitarian Behavior: Does Gender Make the Difference?," *PLoS One* 5, no. 1 (2010): e8865, https://doi.org/10.1371/journal.pone.0008865.

11. Jena McGregor, "The Rundown on Mary Barra, First Female CEO of General Motors," *Washington Post*, December 10, 2013, https://www.washingtonpost.com/news/on-leadership/wp/2013 /12/10/the-rundown-on-mary-barra-first-female-ceo-of-general -motors/.

12. "Discovering the Glass Cliff: Insights into Addressing Subtle Gender Discrimination in the Workplace," University of Exeter, accessed November 19, 2020, http://psychology.exeter.ac.uk /impact/theglasscliff/.

13. Joann Muller, "Exclusive: Inside New CEO Mary Barra's Urgent Mission to Fix GM," *Forbes*, June 16, 2014, https://www.forbes.com /sites/joannmuller/2014/05/28/exclusive-inside-mary-barras-urgent -mission-to-fix-gm/#7427e841c3a5.

Chapter 2: The Risk-Taking Brain

1. "The Beast," Spartan, accessed October 19, 2020, https://race .spartan.com/en/obstacle-course-races/beast.

2. Eden Kendall, in discussion with the author, January 2020.

3. Thekla Morgenroth et al., "Sex, Drugs, and Reckless Driving: Are Measures Biased Toward Identifying Risk-Taking in Men?," *Social Psychological and Personality Science* 9, no. 6 (August 1, 2018): 744–53, https://doi.org/10.1177/1948550617722833.

4. James P. Byrnes, David C. Miller, and William D. Schaefer, "Gender Differences in Risk-Taking: A Meta-Analysis," *Psychological Bulletin* 125, no. 3 (May 1999): 367–83, https://doi.apa.org/doiLanding?doi=10 .1037%2F0033-2909.125.3.367.

5. Sydney Lupkin, "The Hidden Costs of Extreme Obstacle Races,"

ABCNews, May 8, 2014, https://abcnews.go.com/Health/hidden
-cost-extreme-obstacle-races/story?id=23625173.

6. Haddon Rabb and Jillian Coleby, "Hurt on the Hill: A Longitudinal
Analysis of Obstacle Course Racing Injuries," *Orthopaedic Journal
of Sports Medicine* 6, no. 6 (June 2018): https://journals.sagepub
.com/doi/10.1177/2325967118779854.

7. Alvin Powell, "Where Runners Go Wrong," *Harvard Gazette*,
February 23, 2016, https://news.harvard.edu/gazette/story/2016
/02/where-runners-go-wrong/.

8. Hannah A. D. Heage and Tobias Loetscher, "Estimating Everyday
Risk: Subjective Judgments Are Related to Objective Risk, Mapping
of Numerical Magnitudes and Previous Experience," *PLoS ONE* 13,
no. 12: e0207356, https://doi.org/10.1371/journal.pone.0207356.

9. Agam Bansal et al., Selfies: A Boon or Bane?," *Journal of Family
Medicine Primary Care* 7, no. 4 (July-August 2018): 828–31, https://
doi.org/10.4103/jfmpc.jfmpc_109_18.

10. George F. Loewenstein et al., "Risk as Feelings," *Psychological Bulletin*
127, no. 2 (2001): 267–86, https://doi.org/10.1037/0033-2909.127.2.267.

11. Eden Kendall, in discussion with the author, January 2020.

12. Christine R. Harris, Michael Jenkins, and Dale Glaser, "Gender
Differences in Risk Assessment: Why Do Women Take Fewer
Risks than Men?," *Judgment and Decision Making* 1, no. 1 (July
2006): 48–63, http://journal.sjdm.org/jdm06016.pdf.

13. Byrnes, Miller, and Schaefer, "Gender Differences in Risk Taking."

14. "Overcoming Obstacles with Rethreaded at The Spartan Race,"
News 4 Jax, February 21, 2020, https://www.news4jax.com/river
-city-live/2020/02/21/overcoming-obstacles-with-rethreaded-at
-the-spartan-race-river-city-live/.

15. "Overcoming Obstacles with Rethreaded at The Spartan Race."

Chapter 3: The Romantic Brain

1. William R. Jankowiak and Edward F. Fischer, "A Cross-Cultural
Perspective on Romantic Love," *Ethnology* 31, no. 2 (April 1992):
149–55, https://doi.org/10.2307/3773618.

2. Jankowiak and Fischer, "A Cross-Cultural Perspective."
3. Jankowiak and Fischer, "A Cross-Cultural Perspective."
4. Jankowiak and Fischer, "A Cross-Cultural Perspective."
5. Ty Tashiro, accessed October 30, 2020, http://tytashiro.com/the
-science-of-happily-ever-after/.
6. Helen Fisher, Arthur Aron, and Lucy L. Brown, "Romantic Love:
An fMRI Study of a Neural Mechanism for Mate Choice," *Journal
of Comparative Neurology* 493, no. 1 (December 2005): 58–62,
https://doi.org/10.1002/cne.20772.
7. Fisher, Aron, and Brown, "Romantic Love."
8. A. Bartels and S. Zeki, "The Neural Basis of Romantic Love,"
Neuroreport 11 (2000): 3829–834.
9. Sea Captain Date, https://www.seacaptaindate.com/about.
10. Fisher, Aron, and Brown, "Romantic Love."
11. Christopher J. Boyce, Alex M. Wood, and Eamonn Ferguson, "For
Better or For Worse: The Moderating Effects of Personality on
the Marriage–Life Satisfaction Link," *Personality and Individual
Differences* 97 (July 2016): 61–66, https://doi.org/10.1016/j.paid.2016
.03.005.

Chapter 4: The Bonding Brain

1. John Barry, Martin Seager, and Belinda Brown, "Gender Differences
in the Association between Attachment Style and Adulthood
Relationship Satisfaction," *New Male Studies* 4, no. 3 (2015): 63–74.
2. Cindy Hazan and Phillip Shaver, "Romantic Love Conceptualized
as an Attachment Process," *Journal of Personality and Social
Psychology* 52, no. 3 (1987): 511–24, https://doi.org/10.1037/0022
-3514.52.3.511.
3. Barry, Seager, and Brown, "Gender Differences."
4. V. Simard, E. Moss, and K. Pascuzzo, "Early Maladaptive Schemas
and Child and Adult Attachment: A 15-Year Longitudinal Study,"
Psychology and Psychotherapy 84, no. 4 (2011): 349–66, https://doi
.org/10.1111/j.2044-8341.2010.02009.x.
5. Karen M. Grewen et al., "Warm Partner Contact Is Related to

Lower Cardiovascular Activity," *Behavioral Medicine* 29, no. 3 (Fall 2003): 123–30, https://doi.org/10.1080/08964280309596065.

6. Hidenobu Sumioka et al., "Huggable Communication Medium Decreases Cortisol Levels," *Scientific Reports* 3, no. 3034 (2013): 1–6, https://doi.org/10.1038/srep03034.

7. Barry, Seager, and Brown, "Gender Differences."

8. Inna Schneiderman et al., "Oxytocin during the Initial Stages of Romantic Attachment: Relations to Couples' Interactive Reciprocity," *Psychoneuroendocrinology* 37, no. 8 (August 2012): 1277–285, https://doi.org/10.1016/j.psyneuen.2011.12.021.

9. Schneiderman et al., "Oxytocin during the Initial Stages."

10. Ruth Feldman et al., "Evidence for a Neuroendocrinological Foundation of Human Affiliation: Plasma Oxytocin Levels across Pregnancy and the Postpartum Period Predict Mother-Infant Bonding," Psychological Science 18, no. 11 (November 2007): 965–70, https://doi.org/10.1111/j.1467-9280.2007.02010.x.

11. Feldman et al., "Evidence for a Neuroendocrinological Foundation."

12. Jane Starr Drinkard, "A Therapist's Advice for Couples Isolating Together," The Cut, April 1, 2020, https://www.thecut.com/2020 /04/couples-therapist-advice-isolating-with-partner.html.

13. Beate Ditzen et al., "Sex-Specific Effects of Intranasal Oxytocin on Autonomic Nervous System and Emotional Responses to Couple Conflict," *Social Cognitive and Affective Neuroscience* 8, no. 8 (December 2013): 897–902, https://doi.org/10.1093/scan/nss083.

14. Bianca P. Acevedo, "Neural Correlates of Long-Term Intense Romantic Love," *Social Cognitive and Affective Neuroscience* 7, no. 2 (February 2012): 145–59, https://doi.org/10.1093/scan/nsq092.

15. A. Aron et al., "Reward, Motivation and Emotion Systems Associated with Early-Stage Intense Romantic Love," *Journal of Neurophysiology* 93 (2005): 327–37.

16. Sandra Murray, John G. Holmes, and Dale Wesley Griffin, "The Benefits of Positive Illusions: Idealization and the Construction of Satisfaction in Close Relationships," *Journal of Personality and*

Social Psychology 70, no. 1 (January 1996): 79–98, http://doi
.org/10.1037/0022-3514.70.1.79.

17. Dirk Scheele, "Oxytocin Modulates Social Distance between Males
and Females," *Journal of Neuroscience* 32, vol. 46 (November 14, 2012):
16074–79, https://doi.org/10.1523/JNEUROSCI.2755-12.2012.

Chapter 5: Liar, Liar, Brain on Fire

1. Tracy Packiam Alloway and Ross G. Alloway, "Working Memory
Across the Lifespan: A Cross-Sectional Approach," *Journal of
Cognitive Psychology* 25, no. 1 (2013): 84–93, https://doi.org/10.10
80/20445911.2012.748027.

2. B. M. DePaulo, "Lying in Everyday Life," *Journal of Personality
and Social Psychology* 70, no. 5 (1996): 979–95, https://doi.org/10
.1037/0022-3514.70.5.979.

3. Neil Garrett et al., "The Brain Adapts to Dishonesty," Nature
Neuroscience 19 (2016): 1727–732, https://doi.org/10.1038/nn.4426.

4. Artur Marchewka, "Sex, Lies and fMRI—Gender Differences in
Neural Basis of Deception," *PLoS ONE* 7, no. 8 (2012): e43076,
https://doi.org/10.1371/journal.pone.0043076.

5. Maryam Kouchi and Laura J. Kray, "'I Won't Let You Down:'
Personal Ethical Lapses Arising from Women's Advocating for
Others," *Organizational Behavior and Human Decision Processes*
147 (July 2018): 147–57, https://doi.org/10.1016/j.obhdp.2018.06.001.

6. DePaulo, "Lying in Everyday Life."

7. University of Granada, "'Pinocchio Effect' Confirmed: When You
Lie, Your Nose Temperature Rises," ScienceDaily, December 3, 2012,
https://www.sciencedaily.com/releases/2012/12/121203081834.htm.

Chapter 6: The Creative Brain

1. Sarah Halstead (@sarahjhalstead), "Segment from All Together
Now LA Telethon," Instagram video, April 28, 2020, https://www
.instagram.com/p/B_h4l7ZBgJ9/.

2. Sarah Halstead, in discussion with the author, March 21, 2020.

3. Devon Proudfoot, Aaron C. Kay, and Christy Z. Koval, "A Gender Bias in the Attribution of Creativity: Archival and Experimental Evidence for the Perceived Association Between Masculinity and Creative Thinking," *Psychological Science* 26, no. 11 (2015): 1751–61, http://doi.org/10.1177/0956797615598739.

4. Sarah Halstead, in discussion with the author, March 21, 2020.

5. Elizabeth A. Gunderson et al., "Parent Praise to 1- to 3-Year-Olds Predicts Children's Motivational Frameworks 5 Years Later," *Child Development* 84, no. 5 (September-October 2013): 1526–541, https://doi.org/10.1111/cdev.12064.

6. Roger E. Beaty et al., "Robust Prediction of Individual Creative Ability from Brain Functional Connectivity," *PNAS* 115, no. 5 (January 30, 2018): 1087–92, https://doi.org/10.1073/pnas.1713532115.

7. Sarah Halstead, in discussion with the author, March 21, 2020.

8. Anna Abraham et al., "Gender Differences in Creative Thinking: Behavioral and fMRI Findings," *Brain Imaging and Behavior* 8 (2014): 39–51, https://doi.org/10.1007/s11682-013-9241-4.

9. Patrick Cox, "This Is Your Brain on Improv," The World, May 24, 2018, https://www.pri.org/stories/2018-05-23/your-brain-improv.

10. Sarah Halstead, in discussion with the author, March 21, 2020.

11. Cox, "This Is Your Brain on Improv."

Chapter 7: The Happy Brain

1. Gretchen Rubin, *The Happiness Project: Or, Why I Spent a Year Trying to Sing in the Morning, Clean My Closets, Fight Right, Read Aristotle, and Generally Have More Fun* (New York: HarperCollins, 2009), 14.

2. James A. Blumenthal, Patrick J. Smith, and Benson M. Hoffmann, "Is Exercise a Viable Treatment for Depression?," *ACSM's Health & Fitness Journal* 16, no. 4 (2012): 14-21, https://doi.org/10.1249/01.FIT.0000416000.09526.eb.

3. Daniel P. Johnson and Mark A. Whisman, "Gender Differences in Rumination: A Meta-Analysis," *Personality and Individual Differences* 55, no. 4 (2013): 367–74, https://doi.org/10.1016/j.paid.2013.03.019.

4. Nathanial M. Lambert, Frank D. Fincham, and Tyler F. Stillman, "Gratitude and Depressive Symptoms: The Role of Positive Reframing and Positive Emotion," *Cognition & Emotion* 26, no. 4 (2012): 615–33, https://doi.org/10.1080/02699931.2011.595393.

5. Brick Johnstone et al., "Relationships among Spirituality, Religious Practices, Personality Factors, and Health for Five Different Faith Traditions," *Journal of Religious Health* 51 (2012): 1017–1041, https://doi.org/10.1007/s10943-012-9615-8.

6. Angela Jones et al., "Relationships between Negative Spiritual Beliefs and Health Outcomes for Individuals with Heterogeneous Medical Conditions," *Journal of Spirituality in Mental Health* 17, no. 2 (2015): 135–52, https://doi.org/10.1080/19349637.2015.1023679.

7. "The Gender Gap in Religion around the World," Pew Research Center, March 22, 2016, https://www.pewforum.org/2016/03/22 /the-gender-gap-in-religion-around-the-world/.

8. "The Gender Gap in Religion."

9. Emma Green, "Gratitude without God," *Atlantic*, November 26, 2014, https://www.theatlantic.com/health/archive/2014/11/the -phenomenology-of-gratitude/383174/.

10. Neal Krause, "Religious Involvement Gratitude, and Change in Depressive Symptoms Over Time," *International Journal for the Psychology of Religion* 19, no. 3 (July 1, 2009): 155–72, https://doi .org/10.1080/10508610902880204.

11. Prathik Kini et al., "The Effects of Gratitude Expression on Neural Activity," *NeuroImage* 128 (2016): 1–10, https://doi.org /10.1016/j.neuroimage.2015.12.040.

12. Kini et al., "The Effects of Gratitude Expression."

13. Kini et al., "The Effects of Gratitude Expression."

14. Blumenthal, Smith, and Hoffmann, "Is Exercise a Viable Treatment?"

15. N. A. Coles, J. T. Larsen, and H. C. Lench, "A Meta-Analysis of the Facial Feedback Literature: Effects of Facial Feedback on Emotional Experience Are Small and Variable," *Psychological Bulletin* 145, no. 6 (2019): 610–51, https://psycnet.apa.org/doiLanding?doi=10.1037 %2Fbul0000194.

Chapter 8: The Generous Brain

1. Owen S. Good, "The Infamous Potato Salad Kickstarter Fulfills Its Final Goal with This Cookbook," Polygon, July 17, 2016, https://www.polygon.com/2016/7/17/12208840/potato-salad-kickstarter-cookbook-zack-danger-brown.
2. Emily Thompson, "Potato Salad Guy and the Prank That Raised $55,000," *Columbus Monthly*, September 9, 2014, https://www.columbusmonthly.com/article/20140909/LIFESTYLE/309099535.
3. Zack Danger Brown, "Potato Salad," Kickstarter, August 16, 2016, https://www.kickstarter.com/projects/zackdangerbrown/potato-salad/.
4. Atellani, "Women on Kickstarter and the Power of Gender in Analytics," Medium, September 19, 2018, https://medium.com/@atellani/women-on-kickstarter-and-the-power-of-gender-in-analytics-f9a73cb7e030.
5. James Andreoni, Eleanor Brown, and Isaac Rischall, "Charitable Giving by Married Couples: Who Decides and Why Does It Matter?," *Journal of Human Resources* 38, no. 1 (Winter 2003): 111–33, https://doi.org/10.3368/jhr.XXXVIII.1.111.
6. James Andreoni and Lise Vesterlund, "Which Is the Fair Sex? Gender Differences in Altruism," *Quarterly Journal of Economics* 116, no. 1 (February 2001): 293–312, https://doi.org/10.1162/003355301556419.
7. M. Parrett, "An Analysis of the Determinants of Tipping Behavior: A Laboratory Experiment and Evidence from Restaurant Tipping," *Southern Economic Journal* 73 (2006): 489–514, https://doi.org/10.2307/20111903.
8. Leonardo Christov-Moore and Marco Lacoboni, "Self-Other Resonance, Its Control and Prosocial Inclinations: Brain–Behavior Relationships," *Human Brain Mapping* 37, no. 4 (April 2016): 1544–558, https://doi.org/10.1002/hbm.23119.

Chapter 9: The Empathy Brain

1. Ron Carucci, "How to Use Radical Candor to Drive Great Results," *Forbes*, March 14, 2017, https://www.forbes.com/sites

/roncarucci/2017/03/14/how-to-use radical-candor-to-drive-great
-results/?sh=466b59124e23.

2. C. Daniel Batson et al., "Immorality from Empathy-Induced
   Altruism: When Compassion and Justice Conflict," *Journal of
   Personality and Social Psychology* 68, no. 6 (1995): 1042–1054,
   https://doi.org/10.1037/0022-3514.68.6.1042.

3. Batson et al., "Immorality from Empathy-Induced Altruism."

4. Paul Bloom, *Against Empathy: The Case for Rational Compassion*
   (New York: HarperCollins, 2016), 96–97.

5. Elena Gomez, in discussion with the author, July 14, 2020.

6. Varun Warrier et al., "Genome-Wide Analyses of Self-Reported
   Empathy: Correlations with Autism, Schizophrenia, and Anorexia
   Nervosa," *Translational Psychiatry* 8, no. 35 (2018), https://doi.org
   /10.1038/s41398-017-0082-6.

7. Warrier et al., "Genome-Wide Analyses of Self-Reported Empathy."

8. Simon Baron-Cohen et al., "The 'Reading the Mind in the Eyes'
   Test Revised Version: A Study with Normal Adults, and Adults
   with Asperger Syndrome or High-Functioning Autism," *Journal
   of Child Psychology and Psychiatry* 42, no. 2 (2001): 241–51,
   https://pubmed.ncbi.nlm.nih.gov/11280420/.

9. Baron-Cohen et al., "The 'Reading the Mind in the Eyes' Test Revised."

10. Kathleen M. Krol, "Epigenetic Dynamics in Infancy and the Impact
    of Maternal Engagement," *Science Advances* 5, no. 10 (October 16,
    2019): eaay0680, https://doi.org/10.1126/sciadv.aay0680.

11. University of North Florida, "New Social Media Study Investigates
    Relationships among Facebook Use, Narcissism and Empathy,"
    ScienceDaily, July 3, 2014, https://www.sciencedaily.com/releases
    /2014/07/140703102510.htm.

12. William A. Gentry, Todd J. Weber, and Golnaz Sadri, "Empathy
    in the Workplace: A Tool for Effective Leadership," Center for
    Creative Leadership, 2016, https://cclinnovation.org/wp-content
    /uploads/2020/03/empathyintheworkplace.pdf.

13. "The World Is Looking at These Young Indian Entrepreneurs to
    Shake Things Up," Rediff.com, November 16, 2017, https://www

.rediff.com/getahead/report/achievers-forbes-30-under-30-class
-of-2018-world-is-waiting-for-these-young-indian-entrepreneurs
-to-shake-things-up/20171116.htm.

14. Harry Weger Jr., Gina R. Castle, and Melissa C. Emmett, "Active Listening in Peer Interviews: The Influence of Message Paraphrasing on Perceptions of Listening Skill," *International Journal of Listening* 24, no. 1 (2010): 34–49, https://doi.org/10.1080/10904010903466311.

15. Sofie L. Valk et al., "Structural Plasticity of the Social Brain: Differential Change after Socio-Affective and Cognitive Mental Training," *Science Advances* 3, no. 10 (October 4, 2017): e1700489, https://doi.org/10.1126/sciadv.1700489.

16. Tracy Alloway, "Facebook Fearless: How Social Media Can Be Good for You," TEDx Talks, December 12, 2016, YouTube video, 10:29, http://bit.ly/TEDxTracyPAlloway.

Chapter 10: The Leader Brain

1. Belinda Parmar, "Can Empathy Really Work in a Business World Dominated by Testosterone?," *Guardian*, June 18, 2014, https://www.theguardian.com/women-in-leadership/2014/jun/18/empathy-secret-revolutionise-business.

2. Parmar, "Can Empathy Really Work?"

3. Ohio State University, "Narcissistic People Most Likely to Emerge as Leaders," ScienceDaily, October 10, 2008, www.sciencedaily.com/releases/2008/10/081007155100.htm.

4. Annebel H. B. De Hoogh, Deanne N. Den Hartog, and Barbora Nevicka, "Gender Differences in the Perceived Effectiveness of Narcissistic Leaders," *Applied Psychology* 64 (2015): 473–98, https://doi.org/10.1111/apps.12015.

5. J. Ehrlinger and D. Dunning, "How Chronic Self-Views Influence (And Potentially Mislead) Estimates of Performance," *Journal of Personality and Social Psychology* 84, no. 1 (2003): 5–17, https://doi.org/10.1037/0022-3514.84.1.5.

6. Katty Kay and Claire Shipman, "The Confidence Gap," *Atlantic*,

Notes

May 2014, https://www.theatlantic.com/magazine/archive/2014/05/the-confidence-gap/359815/.

7. Amy J. C. Cuddy, Caroline A. Wilmuth, and Dana R. Carney, "The Benefit of Power Posing Before a High-Stakes Social Evaluation," Harvard Business School Working Paper, No. 13-027, September 2012, https://dash.harvard.edu/handle/1/9547823.

8. D. Casasanto, "Embodiment of Abstract Concepts: Good and Bad in Right- and Left-Handers," *Journal of Experimental Psychology: General* 138, no. 3 (2009): 351–67, https://doi.org/10.1037/a0015854.